A Clinical Manual of Pediatric Infectious Disease

Appleton Clinical Manuals

Ayres, et al.: Medical Resident's Manual, 4th edition
Chung: A Clinical Manual of Cardiovascular Medicine
Crain and Gershel: A Clinical Manual of Emergency
Pediatrics
Ellis and Beckmann: A Clinical Manual of Gynecology
Ellis and Beckmann: A Clinical Manual of Obstetrics
Gomella, et al.: Clinician's Pocket Reference, 4th edition
Hanno and Wein: A Clinical Manual of Urology
Matthews, et al.: A Clinical Manual of Adverse Drug
Reactions
Walker and Margouleff: A Clinical Manual of
Nuclear Medicine

A Clinical Manual of Pediatric Infectious Disease

Russell W. Steele, M.D.
Professor of Pediatrics
Division of Infectious Disease/Immunology
University of Arkansas for Medical Sciences and
Arkansas Children's Hospital
Little Rock, Arkansas

 APPLETON-CENTURY-CROFTS/Norwalk, Connecticut

0-8385-1171-6

Copyright © 1986 by Appleton-Century-Crofts
A Publishing Division of Prentice-Hall

86 87 88 89 90 / 10 9 8 7 6 5 4 3 2

Prentice-Hall of Australia, Pty. Ltd., Sydney
Prentice-Hall Canada, Inc.
Prentice-Hall Hispanoamericana, S.A., Mexico
Prentice-Hall of India Private Limited, New Delhi
Prentice-Hall International (UK) Limited, London
Prentice-Hall of Japan, Inc., Tokyo
Prentice-Hall of Southeast Asia (Pte.) Ltd., Singapore
Whitehall Books Ltd., Wellington, New Zealand
Editora Prentice-Hall do Brasil Ltda., Rio de Janeiro

Library of Congress Cataloging in Publication Data
Main entry under title:
Clinical manual of pediatric infectious disease.
   Includes index.
   1. Communicable diseases in children—Handbooks,
manuals, etc.   I. Steele, Russell W., 1942–
[DNLM: 1. Communicable Diseases—in infancy & childhood
—handbooks.   WC 39 C6416]
RJ401.C55 1986   618.92'9   85-13348
ISBN 0-8385-1171-6

Contributors

Watson Arnold, M.D.
Associate Professor of Pediatrics
Director of Pediatric Nephrology

Robert W. Arrington, M.D.
Associate Professor of Pediatrics
Chief, Neonatology

Helen L. Butler, M.D.
Assistant Professor of Pediatrics
Director of Pediatric Gastroenterology

Debra H. Fiser, M.D.
Assistant Professor of Pediatrics and Anesthesiology
Chief of Pediatric Critical Care Medicine

Donald E. Hill, M.D.
Professor of Pediatrics and Physiology
Medical Director of UAMS Nurseries

Richard F. Jacobs, M.D.
Associate Professor of Pediatrics
Division of Infectious Diseases/Immunology

Daniel J. Marmer, M.S.
MT Research Associate

Daniel L. Mollitt, M.D.
Assistant Professor of Pediatrics and Surgery

J. B. Norton, Jr., M.D.
Professor of Pediatrics
Director of Pediatric Cardiology

Richard I. Readinger, M.D.
Assistant Professor of Pediatrics
Pediatric Cardiology

Russell W. Steele, M.D.
Professor of Pediatrics
Division of Infectious Disease/Immunology

Paul C. Stillwell, M.D.
Assistant Professor of Pediatrics
Critical Care Medicine and Pediatric Pulmonology

Joanne S. Szabo, M.D.
Assistant Professor of Pediatrics
Neonatology

Bonnie J. Taylor, M.D.
Assistant Professor of Pediatrics
Neonatology

Becky J. Williams, M.D.
Assistant Professor of Pediatrics
Neonatology

Robert C. Woody, M.D.
Assistant Professor of Neurology and Pediatrics

Terry Yamauchi, M.D.
Professor of Pediatrics
Chief, Pediatric Infectious Diseases

All from the University of Arkansas for Medical Sciences and
Arkansas Children's Hospital, Little Rock, Arkansas

Contents

Preface

Physicians are expected to maintain, at their command, an extensive fund of knowledge. It is, of course, not realistic to commit all important information to memory or even to retain what would be considered essential aspects of diagnosis and treatment. We all, therefore, rely on reference sources for optimal patient care. Our personal libraries not only assure against omissions in medical management but also allow the most efficient method for keeping abreast of new developments in each subspecialty.

In the care of pediatric patients, infectious diseases make up over half of diagnostic considerations. For this reason, the pediatrician or primary care physician who treats children, must particularly prepare him- or herself with a basic understanding of infectious processes. In many cases, knowledge of the disease must be applied in the clinical setting with minimal delay. These situations might be handled best if the physician has at hand a reliable and concise manual that condenses essential information related to diagnosis and treatment. In many cases this may simply offer a rapid check of already planned management. In other cases it may give guidance in an area less familiar to the clinician.

This manual was designed to provide quick reference in the broad area of pediatric infectious diseases. It can be kept in the physician's white coat pocket and the essentials of each topic can be read in just a few minutes. Most information is in tabular or protocol form. The major efforts deal with diagnosis and treatment rather than pathophysiology. The latter should be reviewed as time permits with other standard texts.

Where there is some difference of opinion, particularly for modalities of treatment, we have often elected to present just one approach. This was done to avoid confusion. Every effort has been made to establish a consensus by reviewing standard texts and current medical journals. Major sources have included the following reference books: *Pediatrics,* edited by A. M. Rudolph, *Textbook of Pediatric Infectious Diseases,* by R. D. Feigin and J. D. Cherry, and *Principles and Practice of Infectious Diseases,* by G. L. Mandell, R. G. Douglas, Jr., and J. E. Bennett.

Russell W. Steele

1

Infectious Disease Emergencies

Botulism
Cardiac Infections
Diphtheria
Encephalitis
Epiglottitis
Guillain-Barré Syndrome
Meningitis
Meningococcemia
Peritonitis
Rabies
Reye's Syndrome
Rocky Mountain Spotted Fever
Septic Shock
Tetanus
Toxic Shock Syndrome

There are some infectious disease presentations that must be diagnosed and treated rapidly to prevent mortality and provide optimal prognosis. In many cases, therapy must be instituted before a diagnosis can be confirmed. These are true emergencies and fortunately only a few such entities are commonly encountered in pediatric patients. Sepsis and meningitis are the two most common. In most cases, only one or two laboratory specimens need to be obtained before treatment is begun. In other instances only supportive therapy is warranted either because specific treatment is not yet available or because eradication of the invading pathogen is unnecessary. Such entities are viral encephalitis (other than herpes simplex virus or varicella zoster virus), Reye's syndrome, Guillain-Barré syndrome, infant botulism, and rabies.

Most infectious disease emergencies should be managed in a well-equipped ICU, at least during the acute phase of illness. By definition, progression of disease may require endotracheal intubation or other specialized support procedures. For this reason, transport to referral medical centers should be considered if local facilities do not include intensive care capabilities.

BOTULISM

Botulism is caused by the ingestion of the organism, *Clostridium botulinum*, or its preformed neurotoxin. There are three forms of disease: food-borne, wound, and infant botulism. The only form commonly seen in pediatrics is infant botulism. Disease in infants is thought to be caused by the release of toxin elaborated from organisms that have gained entry into the GI tract.

TABLE 1–1. INFANT BOTULISM: CLINICAL DIAGNOSIS

Symptoms	Physical Findings
Constipation	Generalized hypotonia
Poor feeding	Absent deep tendon reflexes
Weak cry	Dilated reactive pupils
Muscle weakness	Poor suck
Floppiness	Decreased to absent gag reflex
Drooping eyelids	Ptosis
Respiratory distress	

The onset of illness is usually between 8 and 11 weeks with a reported range of 1 week to 10 months. Constipation is the first indication of disease with additional neurologic signs beginning a few days later. The diagnosis is best confirmed by the identification of botulinal toxin in the stool. Culture of the stool for *C. botulinum* should also be attempted but because the organism is ubiquitous, it is not unusual to find this as normal flora in an infant's intestinal tract. The toxin has rarely been observed in the serum of infantile cases although the presence of toxin is fairly consistent in cases of food poisoning and wound botulism.

TABLE 1-2. INFANT BOTULISM: LABORATORY DIAGNOSIS

Toxin in the stool is diagnostic
Stool culture for *C. botulinum*
Electromyography with repetitive stimulation
Lumbar puncture to rule out other diagnoses

The differential diagnosis is rather limited. A lumbar puncture should be performed to rule out other infectious etiologies. A negative response to edrophonium (Tensilon), 1 mg IV or 2 mg IM, and electromyographic studies will differentiate myasthenia gravis.

TABLE 1-3. INFANT BOTULISM: DIFFERENTIAL DIAGNOSIS

Guillain-Barré syndrome
Myasthenia gravis
Sepsis
Aseptic meningitis
Encephalitis
Polio
Diphtheria
Tick paralysis

Treatment is primarily supportive. Antibiotics or antitoxin have not been shown to alter the clinical course. Aminoglycosides should be avoided because these agents can potentiate the neuro-muscular blockade.

TABLE 1-4. INFANT BOTULISM: TREATMENT

Supportive
    Monitor cardiac and respiratory function
    Endotracheal intubation and assisted ventilation
Avoid aminoglycosides

Specific factors predisposing to infant botulism remain specula-tive. A practical approach to prevention, however, might best focus on methods of reducing exposure to spores, which the in-fant might ingest.

TABLE 1-5. INFANT BOTULISM: PREVENTION

Infants < 1 yr of age
    Wash objects placed in infants' mouths (pacifiers, toys, etc.)
    Wash or peel skin of fruits and vegetables
    Avoid honey

CARDIAC INFECTIONS

Infections of the heart in children generally present as life-threat-ening disease requiring management by a pediatric cardiologist. Endocarditis and pericarditis are more commonly caused by bac-terial agents, whereas myocarditis is more likely to have a viral etiology.

TABLE 1-6. ENDOCARDITIS

Etiology
    Bacterial: *Staphylococcus aureus, S. epidermidis, Streptococcus viridans, S. pneumoniae, Enterococcus*
    Other: ARF, SLE, i.e., Libman-Sacks syndrome

TABLE 1-6. (continued)

Clinical
    Underlying congenital or valvular heart defect
      (neonate-associated central hyperalimentation lines)
    Presents slowly over weeks to months with fever, malaise, fatigue
      (occasionally acute with febrile illness, toxicity, CHF)
    Associated findings of ARF or SLE
    Examination: prominent murmur (may have new murmur,
      usually valve insufficiency), findings of CHF
        Embolic findings: petechiae, Roth's spots, Osler's nodes,
        splinter hemorrhages, Janeway lesions, embolic pneumonias,
        splenomegaly
    Chest x-ray: may show enlarged heart or embolic pneumonias
    ECG: nonspecific (ARF may have increased PR interval)
    Laboratory: bacterial endocarditis, positive blood culture, anemia,
      elevated WBC count, left shift, elevated sedimentation rate
      (sedimentation rate may be low with CHF), increased, acute
      phase reactants, RA-positive (80%), ARF (Jones
      criteria), anemia, elevated acute phase reactants, WBC,
      sedimentation rate associated with ASO or streptozyme
    Echo: vegetations on valves or chambers
Course
    Treatment requires specific antibiotic therapy for 6 wk (if cultures
      are negative; semi-synthetic penicillin and aminoglycoside are
      appropriate, acute aortic insufficiency with CHF usually requires
      surgery)
    ARF—3–6 wk aspirin therapy (antiinflammatory levels) and
      bicillin prophylaxis; with severe carditis or CHF—short course
      of steroids is necessary

TABLE 1-7. MYOCARDITIS

Etiology
    Viral: Coxsackie, ECHO, polio, influenzae, adenovirus, mumps,
      rubella
    Bacterial: *S. aureus*, *Neisseria meningitidis*, *Corynebacterium
      diphtheria* (toxin), *Rickettsia rickettsii* (Rocky Mountain Spotted
      Fever)
    Other: ARF (pancarditis), Kawasaki, toxic, parasitic
Clinical
    Febrile illness followed by shortness of breath, malaise, fatigue
      over several weeks to months, may present as an arrhythmia or

(continued)

TABLE 1-7. (continued)

with a fulminant course (especially in young infants) or with
sudden collapse (sudden death), often associated with
pericarditis (myopericarditis)
Bacterial and rickettsial: fulminant illness with sepsis, shock and
CHF
ARF-associated findings (Jones criteria) and findings of valvulitis
(pancarditis)
Kawasaki—acute phase associated with myocarditis and small
vessel arteritis
Examination: findings of CHF
Laboratory
Chest x-ray: enlarged heart (left atrium and ventricle), pulmonary
edema
ECG: diffuse ST–T changes, low voltage, arrhythmias, LVH with
strain pattern (late)
Laboratory: acute phase reactants helpful only early in illness,
laboratory studies for rheumatic or Kawasaki helpful but
nonspecific; viral cultures usually negative
Echo: enlarged LA and LV, poor contractility
MUGA scan: decreased ejection fraction
Gallium scan: increased uptake
Endomyocardial biopsy: diagnostic
Course
Variable course: may show spontaneous improvement with time
or progress to chronic cardiomyopathy
Bacterial and rickettsial (RMSF) etiology have a severe course
with high mortality and need early diagnosis and appropriate
antibiotic coverage
Treatment: supportive, digitalis and diuretics, afterload reducing
agents
Use of steroids and immunosuppressive agents may be helpful if
biopsy or Gallium scan suggest inflammation.

TABLE 1-8. PERICARDITIS

Etiology
Viral: Coxsackie, ECHO, adenovirus, influenza, mumps, EBV
Bacterial: *Haemophilus influenzae, S. aureus, S. pneumoniae, N.
meningitidis*
Other: Uremic, postpericardiotomy, collagen vascular (SLE,
ARF), mycoplasma, TB, parasitic

TABLE 1-8. (continued)

Clinical
   Chest pain, precordial, referred to back and shoulder, relieved by
      sitting up
   Dyspnea
   Fever, malaise (bacterial etiology—increased toxicity)
   Young infant (presents as sepsis associated with meningitis, septic
      arthritis)
   Examination: tachycardia, decreased heart sounds, rub,
      Kussmaul's sign (distention of neck veins with inspiration),
      paradoxical pulse > 10 mm Hg (early tamponade)
   Associated illnesses: renal failure, previous heart surgery, SLE,
      JRA, ARF, meningitis, pneumonia
Laboratory
   Chest x-ray: enlarged, water bottle shaped heart (initially may
      show just a straightened left heart border)
   ECG: diffuse ST–T changes, low voltage
   Laboratory: elevated WBC count, left shift, elevated
      sedimentation rate, renal and collagen vascular studies, blood
      cultures
   Echo: diagnostic
   Pericardial fluid: exudate—protein >3 g/100 ml, cells—many,
      inflammatory (bacterial PMNs), glucose—low, SG >1.015
   Transudate—protein <2 g/100 ml, cells—few (mesothelial),
      glucose—normal, SG <1015
Course
   Bacterial etiology: requires adequate drainage (repeated
      pericardiocentesis or tube drainage), most patients have
      organism recovered via blood or pericardial fluid; appropriate
      antibiotic 14–21 days
   Viral etiology: 2–6 wk, pain usually controlled with aspirin or
      nonsteroidal antiinflammatory drugs (use of steroids
      controversial); viral cultures usually negative, can progress
      occasionally to constriction; tamponade requires
      pericardiocentesis
   Other etiologies: usually follows course of other illness unless
      tamponade occurs

DIPHTHERIA

Diphtheria, an acute illness caused by the organism *Corynebacterium diphtheriae*, is relatively rare in the United States but is still
occasionally seen among the unimmunized population. The incu-

bation period for diphtheria ranges from 1 to 6 days and may present in a number of clinical forms. Because of these various presentations, a wide list of possibilities must be considered in the differential diagnosis.

The diagnosis is confirmed by culture of the material from beneath the pharyngeal membrane. Treatment, however, must be instituted based on clinical suspicion rather than waiting for culture results. The treatment prescribed varies with the severity of the disease as well as duration of the symptoms prior to starting treatment. Prognosis depends on the age of the patient, the location and extent of the membrane, and the promptness with which antitoxin is given.

Consideration must also be given to other persons exposed to the index case; treatment varies with the immune status of the individual.

TABLE 1-9. TREATMENT OF DIPHTHERIA

Antitoxin	Dilute 1:20 in isotonic sodium chloride and infuse IV at rate not to exceed 1 ml/min
Duration under 48 hr and mild symptoms	Dose: 40,000 U
Duration longer than 3 days or severe symptoms	Dose: 80,000 U
Extremely severe or malignant diphtheria	Dose: 100,000–120,000 U
Diphtheria toxoid	First dose: end of 1st wk of illness Second dose: 1 mo later Third dose: 1 mo after the second dose
Antibiotics	Penicillin (100,000 U/kg/day) or erythromycin (20–50 mg/kg/day) × 10 days IV div q6h
Supportive intensive care	Airway protection with endotracheal intubation as needed to assure patent airway and to prevent aspiration

TABLE 1-9. (continued)

Mechanical ventilation for respiratory failure associated with paralysis of muscles of respiration
Support the failing circulation
Bedrest for minimum of 2–3 wk until risk of myocarditis is past
Prednisone 1–1.5 mg/kg/day × 2 wk for myocarditis
Provision for nutrition and hydration via gavage or parenterally, if necessary
Isolation after completion of antibiotic therapy until three cultures of nose and throat (taken 24 hr apart) are negative for toxigenic diphtheria bacilli

TABLE 1-10. MANAGEMENT OF CONTACTS OF INDEX CASES

Immunized household contacts	Schick test, observation
Unimmunized household contacts	Benzathine penicillin 1.2 million U IM or erythromycin 40 mg/kg/day PO × 7 days
	Culture before and after treatment
	Begin diphtheria toxoid immunization
	Observation daily for 7 days

ENCEPHALITIS

Encephalitis is a disorder of cerebral function (an encephalopathy) caused by infection or inflammatory reaction in the CNS.

TABLE 1-11. SIGNS AND SYMPTOMS
OF ENCEPHALITIS

Fever	Delirium
Headache	Convulsions
Irritability	Meningismus
Nausea and vomiting	Focal neurologic signs
Upper respiratory symptoms	Enuresis
Lethargy, stupor	Encopresis

The differential diagnosis of encephalitis includes other causes of encephalopathy.

TABLE 1-12. DIFFERENTIAL DIAGNOSIS OF ACUTE
ENCEPHALOPATHY

Infection
  Meningoencephalitis
  Brain abscess
  Non-CNS infection (e.g., *Shigella*)
Traumatic
  Contusion
  Hemorrhage
Spontaneous hemorrhage
  Aneurysm
  Arterial-venous malformation
Thromboembolism
Vasculitis
Toxic ingestion
Mass effect
  Tumor
  Hemorrhage or effusion
  Cyst
Hydrocephalus
Reye's syndrome
Metabolic disorder
  Uremia
  Hepatic encephalopathy
  Inborn error of metabolism
  Water intoxication
  Hyponatremia
Anoxic encephalopathy

In determining the cause of encephalitis, a number of historic questions may be helpful.

TABLE 1-13. HISTORIC QUESTIONS OF IMPORTANCE IN ENCEPHALITIS

Exposure to illnesses in other humans
Exposure to vectors such as ticks or mosquitoes
Exposure to animals, especially sick animals such as horses
Recent travel
Recent injections
Exposure to environmental toxins

The diagnosis of encephalitis requires examination of the CSF and, cultures of blood, feces, throat, and CSF, and possibly immunologic methods for specific virus identification. Additional information may be gained from EEG, CT, or brain scan, and brain biopsy. With the exception of herpes simplex, the treatment of encephalitis is supportive. Acyclovir has now proven useful as a specific antiviral agent in herpes simplex encephalitis.

TABLE 1-14. DIAGNOSIS OF ENCEPHALITIS

CSF	Smears and cultures for bacteria
	Viral cultures
	Smears and cultures for acid-fast bacteria
	Special preparations for fungi and protozoa
	Leukocyte count (up to several thousand cells, frequently PMN predominance in early stages)
	Protein normal or moderately elevated
	Glucose normal
Blood, feces and throat	Viral cultures
	Immunologic methods
	Detection of viral antigen
	Detection of specific antibodies
EEG	
CT scan	
Radionuclide brain scan	
Brain biopsy	

TABLE 1–15. TREATMENT OF ENCEPHALITIS

Supportive intensive care	Assess airway with regard to adequacy of gas exchange as well as risk of aspiration (patients without purposeful response to pain; comatose); endotracheal intubation as needed for airway protection; mechanical ventilator support as needed to correct hypoventilation or hypoxemia
	Treatment of cerebral edema with resultant increased intracranial pressure: mannitol (0.25 g/kg IV over 30 min), control hyperpyrexia, fluid restriction
	Anticonvulsants as needed for seizure control
	Careful observation for and treatment of fluid and electrolyte imbalances, particularly Syndrome of Inappropriate Antidiuretic Hormone Secretion; hourly monitoring of urine output via bladder catheter
	Chest physiotherapy and tracheal suctioning; frequent turning; range of motion exercises to prevent contractures
	Prophylaxis for stress ulcers or gastritis with antacid therapy, preferably guided by measurement of gastric pH
Specific antiviral therapy	For herpes simplex encephalitis (diagnosed on brain biopsy): Acylovir 30 mg/kg/day IV div q8h × 10 days

EPIGLOTTITIS

Acute epiglottitis is a life-threatening form of acute upper airway obstruction. It is almost always caused by *Haemophilus influenzae* infection, though other organisms have rarely been cultured. Affecting predominately young children under 4 years of age, epiglottitis presents an acutely toxic appearance of sudden onset.

**TABLE 1-16. SIGNS AND SYMPTOMS OF
EPIGLOTTITIS AT TIME OF HOSPITAL ADMISSION**

Sign or Symptom	% of Patients
Respiratory distress	100
Stridor	92
Fever	92
Drooling	63
Delirium	58
Dysphagia	58
Pharyngitis	50
Hoarseness	33
Cough	29

The diagnosis is made from the characteristic clinical presentation in most cases. In severe or classic cases, nothing is gained by waiting for a lateral neck radiograph to confirm the diagnosis; a patent airway must be established as rapidly as possible. On the other hand, this examination may provide useful information in the patient with mild symptoms in whom the diagnosis of croup is being considered. In the event that radiographic examination is elected, the physician should accompany the patient at all times. Acute epiglottis must be differentiated from other disorders producing supraglottic and subglottic upper airway obstruction.

TABLE 1-17. DIFFERENTIAL DIAGNOSIS

Croup
Peritonsillar abscess
Retropharyngeal abscess
Severe tonsillitis
Foreign body aspiration
Angioedema
Infectious mononucleosis

Once the diagnosis of epiglottitis is seriously suspected, preparations must begin immediately to secure the airway. When treated early and aggressively, the prognosis for epiglottitis is excellent.

TABLE 1-18. TREATMENT OF EPIGLOTTITIS

Secure airway	Keep child calm, preferably in parent's arms
	Administer oxygen by face mask if possible without agitating the child
	Contact anesthesiologist, otolaryngologist, and operating room supervisor
	Transport as soon as possible to operating room accompanied by parent (to calm child), physician, and all equipment needed to secure airway if distress increases in transport
	Induce anesthesia by allowing child to breathe spontaneously from mask halothane and 100% oxygen while in sitting position; then, establish IV line
	The epiglottis is visualized for direct examination and a nasotracheal tube is inserted, if possible. (In cases where this is not possible, orotracheal intubation is attempted, followed by bronchoscopic intubation, or finally tracheostomy as a last resort.) The tube is taped securely in place with a strip all the way around the back of the child's head
	Obtain blood cultures after airway is secure
Antibiotics	Cefotaxime, ceftizoxime, ceftriaxone, moxalactam, or chloramphenicol
Supportive care	Observe in ICU; keep sedated and restrained; provide 2 cm H_2O CPAP and humidification to endotracheal tube; assure hydration intravenously
Extubation	After approximately 48 hr intubation, the epiglottis is again examined directly; if edema and inflammation have subsided, the tube may be removed; if not, the tube is left in place and the epiglottis is reexamined in 24 hr

GUILLAIN-BARRÉ SYNDROME (GBS)

GBS (acute idiopathic polyneuritis) is one of the most serious pediatric neurologic disorders. Although the majority of cases of GBS are mild and self-limited, at times the disorder may progress to complete respiratory paralysis and severe autonomic dysfunction. The overall incidence is 1 to 2 cases per 100,000 population. Although the disorder most frequently occurs in the winter and spring months, it may occur at any time of the year.

The underlying pathology of GBS is nearly symmetrical demyelination of the peripheral nervous system segmentally from the ventral and dorsal root ganglia distally. Lymphocytic and macrophagic infiltration is characteristic, although the mechanism leading to this infiltration is not fully understood.

TABLE 1-19. FACTORS ASSOCIATED WITH THE ONSET OF GBS

Infectious or postinfectious factors (60%)
  Viral
    Nonspecific upper respiratory or GI
    EBV
    CMV
  Rickettsia
  Mycoplasma
  Bacterial
Noninfectious factors (10%)
  Vaccination
  Immune disorders
  Endocrine disturbances
  Pregnancy
  Neoplasms
  Toxic exposures
  Surgery

The clinical presentation of GBS is notoriously variable. The classic case includes an ascending paralysis with sensory symptoms such as muscle cramps with few sensory signs. GBS may present, however, atypically with a descending paralysis, ophthalmoplegia, or a "locked-in" state with complete motor paralysis in which the patient appears comatose.

TABLE 1-20. DIAGNOSTIC CRITERIA OF GBS

Criteria required for diagnosis
  Progressive motor weakness of more than one limb and/or truncal or bulbar weakness
  Areflexia
Criteria strongly suggestive of the diagnosis
  Minimal sensory findings
  Relative symmetry of weakness
  Progressive motor involvement of 2-4 wk followed by a plateau and gradual complete recovery
  Cranial nerve involvement, especially bifacial paralysis
  Autonomic system involvement
  Absence of fever at onset
  Elevated CSF protein at some point during illness
  CSF cell count < 10 mononuclear cells/ml^3
  Nerve conduction velocities slowed or blocked and possibly prolonged distal latencies at some point during the illness
Factors inconsistent with the diagnosis
  Marked asymmetry of weakness
  Persistent bowel or bladder dysfunction
  Sudden onset of bowel or bladder dysfunction
  Greater than 50 mononuclear cells/ml^3 or the presence of any polymorphonuclear leukocytes in CSF
  Sharp sensory level
Factors that exclude the diagnosis
  History of toxic hydrocarbon or lead exposure, acute intermittent porphyria, diphtheria, botulism, poliomyelitis, or other well recognized causes of neuropathies.
  Purely sensory symptoms

The natural history of severe GBS may be altered by early recognition and the availability of intensive care, in particular, ventilatory support. With such support, all children with GBS should survive with a favorable outcome. The most common pediatric complications of GBS are respiratory arrest, aspiration pneumonia, complications of autonomic dysfunction, and iatrogenic complications of prolonged ventilation.

TABLE 1-21. THE NATURAL HISTORY OF GBS

20% require ventilatory support
5-10% relapse
50% make complete recovery
10% have residual neurologic or orthopedic sequelae
5% die of pulmonary or cardiac (adults) complications

The management of children with GBS requires physicians, nurses, respiratory therapists, and physical and occupational therapists who are acquainted with the natural history and evolution of the disorder. In general, any patient with suspected GBS should be admitted to a pediatric ICU or a ward in which meticulous observation and neurologic reexamination is possible. GBS may acutely evolve from minimal motor weakness to complete respiratory paralysis in some cases.

TABLE 1-22. MANAGEMENT OF GBS

Chronic neurologic care
   Prevention of UTI
   Prevention of decubiti
   Prevention of immobilization hypercalcemia and renal or bladder
    calculi
   Prevention of contractures
   Recognition and treatment (in some cases) of autonomic
    dysfunction
Respiratory care
   Admission to ICU setting
   Recognition of deteriorating respiratory ability through clinical
    observation, pulmonary function tests, and/or ABG analysis;
    endotracheal intubation and mechanical ventilation as needed
    for respiratory failure
   Vigorous treatment of pulmonary infections
   Tracheostomy when mechanical ventilation is prolonged
Potential pharmacologic management of GBS
   Corticosteroids: no proven efficacy in acute GBS
   Treatment of autonomic dysfunction: rarely indicated
      Antihypertensives (diuretic agents)
      Fluorocortisone (Florinef) for marked orthostatic hypotension
      Plasmapheresis (controlled studies under way)

The pharmacologic treatment of GBS remains in question. Corticosteroid therapy has not been proven to be of efficacy in GBS. The use of immunosuppressants, such as azothioprine or cyclophosphamide has not been shown in controlled studies to be efficacious and plasmapheresis is currently being evaluated in controlled studies.

MENINGITIS

Bacterial meningitis is a common cause for hospitalization in ICUs. The diagnosis is usually made by examination of the CSF in the child who presents with clinical signs of sepsis, particularly with physical signs localizing that infection to the CNS, i.e., irritability, lethargy, meningismus. The absence of these physical findings, however, does not rule out meningitis, particularly in the young infant. Meningitis should be suspected and sought in infants with fever, lethargy, irritability, and/or poor feeding. The clinician's assessment of the degree of "toxicity" of the child has proven to be the most valuable tool in identifying the child with possible meningitis.

TABLE 1–23. ETIOLOGY OF BACTERIAL MENINGITIS

Neonatal
   Group B streptococcus
   Escherichia coli
   Listeria monocytogenes
   Group D streptococcus
   Gram-negative coliforms
   Staphylococcus aureus
Older child
   Haemophilus influenzae
   Neisseria meningitidis
   Streptococcus pneumoniae

Management includes antibiotics as well as observation and treatment for any secondary complications that may occur.

TABLE 1-24. MANAGEMENT OF MENINGITIS

Initial evaluation
    Lumbar puncture
    Blood culture
    CBC, platelet count
    Electrolytes (SIADH)
    BUN (dehydration)
    Creatinine
    Glucose (hypoglycemia, comparison to CSF glucose)
    ABG
Inpatient
    Chest x-ray
    PT
    Liver enzymes and bilirubin
    Serum (to hold)
    Urinalysis
Supportive care
    Monitor (BP, fluid balance, neurologic and cardiac examinations)
    Restrict fluids to 3-4 of maintenance
    Anticonvulsants for seizures
Antibiotics (for dosages see Tables 18–10 and 18–12)
    Neonate (birth to 3 mo): ampicillin *PLUS*
      cefotaxime, ceftriaxone, moxalactam, or gentamicin
Infants and children (>3 mo): ceftriaxone (alone), cefotaxime
    (alone), or moxalactam + penicillin
Laboratory monitoring
    HCT daily
    CBC weekly
    Electrolytes as indicated (SIADH)
    Renal and liver function as indicated
    Urine sodium, osmolality (SIADH)
    Antibiotic drug levels (aminoglycosides or chloramphenicol)
    CSF: 24–48 hr into therapy
    Ultrasound or CT scan when indicated
Outpatient follow-up
    2 wk: auditory testing
         head circumference
         neurologic examination
    6 wk, 3 mo, 1 yr: neurologic examination

A variety of problems may complicate the course of meningitis in both the early phase of the disease and chronically.

TABLE 1-25. COMPLICATIONS OF BACTERIAL MENINGITIS

Early
    Deafness
    Cerebral edema
    Seizures
    SIADH
    Cranial nerve palsies
    Shock
    Disseminated intravascular coagulation
    Myocarditis
    Pericarditis
    Endocarditis
    Subdural effusion
    Brain abscess
Late
    Hydrocephalus
    Cranial nerve palsies (including deafness and blindness)
    Paralysis
    Mental retardation
    Muscular hypertonia
    Seizures

Prophylaxis of household and day-care nursery contacts of index cases of meningococcal and *H. influenzae* meningitis is discussed in Chapter 3.

TABLE 1-26. PROPHYLAXIS FOR FAMILY CONTACTS OF INDEX CASES OF *H. INFLUENZAE* OR MENINGOCOCCAL MENINGITIS

Rifampin
	Adults	600 mg/day div qd × 4 days
	Children	
	>1 mo	20 mg/kg/day div qd × 4 days
	<1 mo	10 mg/kg/day div qd × 4 days

MENINGOCOCCEMIA

The organism *Neisseria meningitidis* causes an illness in humans
with a variety of clinical presentations ranging from benign upper
respiratory infection to acute endotoxemia and vasculitis to
chronic disease. The common signs and symptoms of acute and
chronic meningococcemia may initially be subtle, but fever accompanied by a petechial rash should always suggest this diagnosis.

The diagnosis of meningococcemia is made with a characteristic clinical presentation and usually is confirmed by culture.

TABLE 1-27. LABORATORY DIAGNOSIS FOR MENINGOCOCCEMIA

CBC—leukocytosis (usually) and thrombocytopenia
Cultures—blood, CSF, skin lesion, nasopharynx
CSF—pleocytosis, elevated protein, low glucose
Counterimmunoelectrophoresis for types A, C, and D
Clotting studies—low PT, fibrinogen, factors V and VIII with DIC
Urinalysis—proteinuria and hematuria

Care must be taken to differentiate meningococcemia from
other febrile illnesses with rash. These include septicemia with
other bacteria, particularly *H. influenzae*, endocarditis, Rocky
Mountain spotted fever, and enteroviral infections.

Treatment includes antibiotics and intensive supportive care
when shock is present. In addition, prophylactic treatment of
family and other close contacts of the index case is indicated
using rifampin.

TABLE 1-28. TREATMENT OF MENINGOCOCCEMIA

Aqueous penicillin G when diagnosis is known (400,000 U/kg/day)
  IV div q6h × 7-10 days
Methylprednisolone 30 mg/kg (maximum of 2 g) IV may be useful

(continued)

TABLE 1-28. (continued)

in shock when given early in the course; repeat dose in 4–8 hr if
  needed
Aggressive fluid resuscitation for the patient in shock to replete
  intravascular volume (see Table 1–53 for supportive care)
Platelet or clotting factor replacement therapy for the patient in
  DIC with hemorrhage
Burn-type wound care for skin sloughs in areas of thrombosis

PERITONITIS

Acute bacterial peritonitis occurs in two distinct forms as determined by the source of infection.

TABLE 1-29. CHARACTERISTICS OF FORMS
OF PERITONITIS

Primary
  Focus is outside the abdominal cavity and the infection is blood–
    or lymphborne; commonly seen in children with ascites
    secondary to nephrosis or cirrhosis
Secondary
  Infection disseminated by extension from or rupture of an
    intraabdominal viscus or abscess of an intraabdominal organ

TABLE 1-30. BACTERIOLOGY OF PERITONITIS

Primary peritonitis
  S. pneumoniae
  Streptococci
  Gram-negative rods
  Mycobacterium tuberculosis
  H. influenzae
Secondary peritonitis
  Aerobic bacteria
  E. coli
  Streptococci
    Enterococci
  S. aureus

TABLE 1-30. (continued)

Enterobacteraciae/*Klebsiella*
   Proteus
   Pseudomonas
 Candida
Anaerobic bacteria
 Bacteroides
   Bacteroides fragilis
 Eubacteria
 Clostridia
 Peptostreptococci
 Peptococci
 Propionibacteria
 Fusobacteria

Peritonitis should be suspected from the clinical presentation and confirmed by laboratory evaluation.

TABLE 1-31. SIGNS AND SYMPTOMS OF GENERALIZED PERITONITIS

Abdominal pain and tenderness
Edema
Ascites
Fever
Anorexia, vomiting, constipation or diarrhea
Ileus
Lethargic, toxic-appearing child
Abdominal wall cellulitis

TABLE 1-32. LABORATORY DIAGNOSIS OF PERITONITIS

Leukocytosis
Radiographic examination of abdomen
  Dilation of large and small intestines

(*continued*)

TABLE 1-32. (continued)

Edema of small intestinal wall
Peritoneal fluid
Obliteration of psoas shadow
Free air in the peritoneal cavity (secondary peritonitis)
Paracentesis (Chap. 5)
  Elevated protein concentration
  Pleocytosis (more than 300 leukocytes/mm^3, more than 25% of
    which are PMN)
Positive Gram smear and culture of fluid

The treatment for bacterial peritonitis is nonoperative for primary peritonitis and operative for secondary peritonitis.

Common postoperative complications include formation of adhesions with subsequent intestinal obstruction and intraabdominal abscess formation.

TABLE 1-33. TREATMENT OF PERITONITIS

Primary
  Systemic antibiotics — Cefotaxime (200 mg/kg/day), ceftriaxone (100 mg/kg/day), or moxalactam (200 mg/kg/day) IV div q6h
Secondary
  Preoperative disturbances — Correction of hypovolemia and electrolyte stabilization to reestablish adequate urine output
  Correction of hypoxemia with supplemental oxygen and mechanical ventilation, if necessary
  Decompression of gastrointestinal tract using nasogastric suction or long intestinal tube
  Antibiotics — Ampicillin (200 mg/kg/day), clindamycin (40 mg/kg/day), and gentamicin (7.5 mg/kg/day) IV div q6h

TABLE 1-33. (continued)

Operative therapy	Close, exclude, or resect perforated viscus
	EITHER complete exposure of peritoneal cavity with radical debridement of peritoneum, followed by massive irrigation with or without antibiotics *OR* placement of drains after repair of perforation without further exploration or irrigation
Postoperative management	Continued administration of systemic antibiotics
	Intraperitoneal lavage with antibiotic solution
	Attention to repletion of intravascular fluid volume
	Nutritional support to meet high metabolic demands
	Close observation for intraabdominal abscess formation

RABIES

Rabies is an acute encephalomyelitis caused by a rhabdovirus. Transmitted via the saliva in the bite of an infected animal, the virus passes along peripheral nerves to the CNS where neuronal necrosis occurs, principally in the brainstem and medulla. The incubation varies from 10 days to as long as 2 years with the mean onset within 2 months after the bite.

TABLE 1-34. FACTORS AFFECTING TIME TO ONSET OF SYMPTOMS

Distance of site of initial inoculum from CNS
Amount of inoculum
Virulence of the virus
Resistance of the host

There are two basic presentations for the disease in humans, classic and paralytic. The classic symptom of hydrophobia is caused by inspiratory muscle spasms that may be due to destruction of the brainstem neurons inhibitory to the neurons of the nucleus ambiguous, which controls inspiration.

TABLE 1-35. SYMPTOMS OF THE CLASSIC FORM OF RABIES

Prodrome	2 days–2 wk	Malaise, anorexia, headache, fever, irritability, pain, numbness or tingling at the site of the bite spreading upward; later, jerky movements, pupillary dilatation, increased tearing and salivation
Acute neurologic phase	2–7 days	Dysphagia, hydrophobia, mania alternating with lethargy, increased salivation, abnormal biting and chewing, excitement, fear, apathy, terror, convulsive movements, choking, distended bladder, constipation, penile pain
Final phase	7–10 days	Coma, dysrhythmias, hypotension, heart block, bradycardia, respiratory muscle spasm, hypoventilation, fluid balance and other metabolic upsets, cardiorespiratory arrest

The diagnosis may be confirmed by demonstration of the antigen, antibody, or viral complexes.

TABLE 1-36. DIAGNOSIS OF RABIES

Identify antigen in cell culture
  Electron microscopy
  Immunofluorescent rabies antibody staining
Antibody titers
  Diagnostic in nonvaccinated persons
  CSF titers used to diagnose postvaccination encephalomyelitis
Viral complexes
  Corneal touch preparations
  Fluorescent antibody in parafollicular neurons of neck skin
   biopsy

The differential diagnosis includes other causes of encephalitis and ascending neuritis.

Prevention of rabies includes measures to control the reservoir animal population as well as vaccination of domestic animals (95% effective). Postexposure treatment of humans includes human rabies immune globulin and human diploid cell vaccine (see Chap. 4). The only sure protection, however, is immunity acquired preexposure.

Once a victim is clinically symptomatic, the prognosis is grim with only extremely rare survivors. Treatment centers on intensive supportive care with aggressive intervention to control the airway and assure optimal ventilation in the patient with hydrophobia or obtundation as well as circulatory system support, the goal being to stabilize the patient until the CNS recovers.

REYE'S SYNDROME

Reye's syndrome is an acute encephalopathy of uncertain etiology. It usually presents within 48 hours of recovery from a previous viral illness, most commonly influenza B or chickenpox. Various toxins have also been implicated as causing a clinical picture similar to Reye's syndrome.

The clinical presentation varies with the age of the child.

TABLE 1–37. CLINICAL PRESENTATION OF REYE'S SYNDROME

Neonatal
  No viral prodrome
  Tachypnea, respiratory
    alkalosis or respiratory
    compensation for metabolic
    acidosis
  Seizures, generalized and
    tonic
  Temperature instability
  Hyperammonemia
Older infant
  Gastroenteritis
  Tachypnea, respiratory
    alkalosis or respiratory
    compensation for metabolic
    acidosis
  Seizures
  Obtundation
  Apnea
  Hepatomegaly
  Hyperammonemia
  Hypoglycemia

Older child
  Viral prodrome
  Intractable vomiting during
    recovery
  Combativeness
  Lethargy
  Confusion
  Irritability
  Decerebrate posturing
  Hyperventilation with
    respiratory alkalosis
  Hepatomegaly and
    hepatocellular dysfunction

Using the clinical assessment of level of consciousness, respiration, and pupillary and oculocephalic reflexes, patients may be categorized by clinical stage.

TABLE 1–38. CLINICAL STAGING OF REYE'S SYNDROME

Stage I	Vomiting, lethargy, irritability, personality changes
Stage II	Disorientation, delirium, combativeness, purposeful response to pain

TABLE 1-38. (continued)

Stage III	Coma, decorticate posturing with painful stimuli, hyperventilation, normal pupillary and oculocephalic reflexes
Stage IV	Deepening coma, decerebrate posturing with painful stimuli, dilated pupils with sluggish reaction to light, lose oculocephalic reflex
Stage V	Flaccidity, apnea, fixed and dilated pupils, only spinal reflexes present

TABLE 1-39. LABORATORY ABNORMALITIES IN REYE'S SYNDROME

Arterial blood ammonia—increased
Serum transaminases—increased
Bilirubin—normal
Fibrinogen—decreased
Prothrombin time—prolonged
Hemoglobin—normal
Platelet count—normal
WBC counts—normal or high
Serum fatty acids—increased
Serum amino acids—elevations of glutamine, proline, alanine, and α amino-N-butyrate
Blood glucose—normal, low, or high
Serum lactic acid—increased
Serum bicarbonate—normal or decreased
EEG—normal or slowing which may progress in severity to electrocerebral silence
CT—normal or diffuse edema
Serum complement—decreased
Creatine phosphokinase muscle isoenzymes—increased

The diagnosis may be confirmed by liver biopsy; however, clinical criteria may be applied to reach a presumptive diagnosis of Reye's syndrome. There are some cases, however, in which the liver biopsy is generally recommended in order to rule out other disease processes.

TABLE 1-40. CRITERIA FOR DIAGNOSIS OF REYE'S SYNDROME

Viral prodrome with compatible clinical history
Normal CSF cell count
Hyperammonemia (150% of normal) and increase in serum
  transaminases (200% of normal)
Exclusion of other causes of encephalopathy and hepatocellular
  dysfunction
Liver biopsy—indications
  Infants
  Children with recurrent episodes
  Familial cases
  Nonepidemic cases without viral prodrome or history of vomiting

TABLE 1-41. DIFFERENTIAL DIAGNOSIS OF REYE'S SYNDROME

Toxic ingestion
Infectious meningitis or encephalitis
Shigellosis
Hepatitis and hepatic coma
Ornithine transcarbamylase deficiency
Systemic carnitine deficiency
Asphyxial encephalopathy and hepatopathy

The treatment of Reye's syndrome is principally supportive with special attention to control of elevated intracranial pressure due to cerebral edema. These measures are generally weaned in reverse order from their institution as the patient improves. In recent years, despite improvements in the prognosis of Reye's syndrome since the institution of protocols for control of intracranial pressure, the metabolic derangement in some patients is so severe that a few patients succumb to the disease despite optimal control of the intracranial pressure.

Treatment

Stage I. Minimize stimulation by placing patient in quiet room.

Position in bed so that head is elevated 30 degrees and positioned in midline to maximize venous drainage from the brain.

Control hyperpyrexia, if present, using cooling blanket, if necessary.

Restrict intake of free water; total fluids limited to 75% of maintenance unless shock is present.

Regulate intravenous glucose infusion to keep blood sugar at approximately 150 mg%.

Supplement oxygen as needed to keep PaO_2 between 100 and 150 mm Hg.

Give vitamin K, 5 mg IM, if prothrombin time is prolonged; double dose if no improvement.

Replace with fresh frozen plasma for clotting factors if there is active hemorrhage.

For hyperammonemia begin lactulose (15–30 ml q4–6h) titrated to keep stool pH less than 7.0.

Antacids: cimetidine (20 mg/kg/day divided in 4 doses); add oral antacid if needed (10–30 ml q2–4h), titrated to keep gastric aspirate pH greater than 3.5

Daily laboratory results (more frequently if indicated by clinical situation): CBC, electrolytes, glucose, BUN, ammonia.

Transfuse with packed red blood cells as needed for anemia (HCT less than 34%) to provide for optimal oxygen delivery to the brain.

Take cultures and prescribe antibiotics if indicated by fever or leukocytosis.

Give attention to nutrition when stable (usually by at least the third hospital day).

Stage II. Continue above measures and add sedation with low doses of pentobarbital (1 mg/kg/dose IV q1–2h), OR morphine (0.005 mg/kg/dose IV q4h), OR lorazepam (0.04 mg/kg IV).

Stages III and IV. Continue above measures and add endotracheal intubation. Use a technique that minimizes iatrogenic increase in intracranial pressure during the procedure. Assemble appropriate equipment to include endotracheal tube, laryngoscope and blade, bag and mask, and suction. Preoxygenate with 100% oxygen by allowing patient to breathe spontaneously from bag and mask for at least 3 minutes. Administer atropine 0.02 mg/kg IV (unless heart rate greater than 150), pentothal 5 mg/kg IV (monitoring for hypotension which may occur in a volume depleted patient), followed by succinylcholine 1.5 mg/kg IV. Perform direct laryngoscopy and intubate using continuous cricoid compression to minimize chances of gastric contents aspiration. Listen for equality of breath sounds and follow with chest radiograph to verify correct tube placement.

Mechanical hyperventilation using tidal volume 12–15 ml/kg, adjusting rate as necessary to lower $PaCO_2$ to 25 mm Hg; supplemental oxygen to keep PaO_2 100–150 mm Hg; CPAP 2–4 cm H_2O to prevent atelectasis; arterial blood gas analysis at least q4–6h; endotracheal suctioning only when needed in order to minimize rises in intracranial pressure; chest physiotherapy is rarely tolerated; daily chest radiographs while intubated.

Establish arterial line preferably in radial artery to allow continuous monitoring of arterial blood pressure and to facilitate arterial blood gas sampling; establish central line for monitoring intravascular volume status (CVP or Swan-Ganz catheter); insert indwelling bladder catheter to allow hourly assessment of urine output. Central lines should be changed or removed if no longer needed after 3 days, arterial lines after 5 days.

Neurosurgical consultation for urgent placement of intracranial pressure monitor. Monitor should be left in place until therapy for control of pressure has all been weaned.

Institute osmotherapy with mannitol 0.25 g/kg q4h as needed for control of intracranial pressure and regulation of serum osmolarity; monitor serum osmolarity at least q8h with adjustments in dose to keep it between 300–320 mOsm/liter.

During therapy, careful attention should be paid to skin care with frequent turning to prevent decubitus ulcers and passive range of motion exercises (if intracranial pressure tolerates) to prevent formation of contractures.

For acute rises in intracranial pressure to level greater than 20 mm Hg with resultant decrease in cerebral perfusion pressure to level less than 50 mm Hg, draw ABG (to rule out hypoxemia or hypercarbia as etiology of acute rise) followed immediately by trial of manual hyperventilation. Also reassess fluid balance to rule out volume overload as etiology of acute rise in pressure.

If intracranial pressure remains poorly controlled, add neuromuscular blockade with Pavulon (0.01 mg/kg/dose q45–60min). Continue sedative as previously described.

If intracranial pressure is still poorly controlled, cool patient to between 32° and 34°C (watching for bradycardia or hypotension due to myocardial depression).

If intracranial pressure is still poorly controlled, institute therapeutic barbiturate coma with pentobarbital using the lowest level of drug necessary to achieve control of intracranial pressure. Institute loading with boluses of 10 mg/kg over 5 to 10 minutes repeated up to two more times until 30 mg/kg total dose has been given OR pressure has been controlled OR patient becomes flaccid and apneic clinically OR electrocortical silence appears on EEG tracing during continuous monitoring OR evidence of hypotension appears necessitating that remainder of loading be delayed until the circulation is stabilized.

During loading, be prepared to deal with hypotension caused by venodilatation (low preload documented by measuring central venous or pulmonary capillary wedge pressure) or by myocardial depression. The treatment of hypotension would include replacement of intravascular volume initially using isotonic crystalloid or colloid solution followed by the use of an inotropic agent, such as dobutamine, infusion 5 to 10 μg/kg/min if needed.

After loading is accomplished, a maintenance IV infusion of pentobarbital should be instituted at a dose 1 mg/kg/hr. Serum levels should be monitored at least q8h because of the cumulative effect of pentobarbital once the fat is saturated. This may result in a sudden precipitous rise in serum concentration without any recent change in dose. At this time it is usually feasible to discontinue administration of the drug completely as levels tend to fall back to normal very slowly over the next 3 to 4 days. As the level falls, loss of control of intracranial pressure may be an indication that pentobarbital infusion should be reinstituted.

Note that both hypothermia and barbiturate therapy may lower metabolism and consequently decrease CO_2 production. It is usually necessary to decrease the number of ventilator breaths the patient receives when these measures are instituted to avoid overventilation using arterial blood gases as a guide.

The clinical evaluation of the patient in therapeutic barbiturate coma becomes unreliable with usually reversible loss of brainstem reflexes, apnea, and flaccidity mimicking brain death. Evaluation of brainstem auditory evoked responses, however, may still be used to demonstrate the intactness of the brainstem during therapy. In addition, it is useful to evaluate the intracranial compliance intermittently to document improvement. This may be assessed clinically by noting the intracranial pressure response to noxious stimuli, suctioning, turning the head to one side, or jugular venous compression.

In addition, close attention must be paid to the potential development of infection while receiving high dose barbiturates as there may be no clinical clues that sepsis is present. Daily blood cultures and urinalyses are recommended.

If intracranial pressure still remains poorly controlled despite the measures outlined above, surgical decompression is recommended by some centers. However, its use remains controversial.

Stage V. Patients presenting with stage V disease may have such severe irreversible brain damage that aggressive measures such as those described above are not warranted.

ROCKY MOUNTAIN SPOTTED FEVER

Rocky Mountain spotted fever is a disease caused by inoculation with *Rickettsia rickettsii* organisms transmitted via the bite of a tick. The organisms replicate within the endothelial lining and smooth muscle cells of blood vessels, causing a generalized vasculitis. The involvement of various organ systems with the vasculitis results in the clinical findings.

TABLE 1–42. CLINICAL FINDINGS IN ROCKY MOUNTAIN SPOTTED FEVER

History of tick bite in 70–80%
Fever
Headache, anorexia, chills, sore throat, nausea and vomiting, abdominal pain, mild diarrhea, arthralgias, and myalgias
Rash: Petechial but may begin as macular or maculopapular; blanching lesions; affects extremities first and spreads centripetally; occasionally appears later or not at all
Noncardiogenic pulmonary edema
Occasional manifestations: edema (periorbital early, then generalized), splenomegaly (present in one-third of cases), hepatomegaly, pneumonitis, myocardial involvement, conjunctivitis, photophobia, papilledema, transient deafness, meningismus, delirium, seizures, coma

The incubation period in children ranges from 1 to 8 days. When the early, nonspecific symptoms appear in a child with a history of a tick bite, Rocky Mountain spotted fever should be seriously considered with early treatment instituted. Most laboratory findings in Rocky Mountain spotted fever are nonspecific until positive convalescent antibody titers appear. The exception to this is the appearance of the organism on stain of skin lesion or the use of immunofluorescent biopsy of skin for early specific diagnosis.

TABLE 1–43. LABORATORY STUDIES IN ROCKY MOUNTAIN SPOTTED FEVER

WBC count—normal or slightly decreased with left shift in first week; leukocytosis second week
Platelet count—depressed

(continued)

TABLE 1-43. (continued)

Fibrinogen—depressed with DIC
Electrolytes—hyponatremia and hypochloremia
Liver function tests—elevated SGOT, SGPT, bilirubin; depressed
  total protein and albumin
Creatinine—increased
LDH—increased
Urinalysis—hematuria
CSF—WBC count $\leq 300/mm^3$, predominately lymphocytes in most
  cases; normal glucose; mildly elevated protein
Weil-Felix reaction—proteus OX-19 and OX-2 single titer $> 1:160$
  or fourfold rise in titer diagnostic
Rocky Mountain spotted fever complement fixation
  titers—convalescent titers may increase after the 14th day of illness
Giemsa stain of skin lesion—may be able to demonstrate organism
Immunofluorescent biopsy of skin—may be possible to make early
  diagnosis using this technique.

It may at times be difficult to differentiate Rocky Mountain
spotted fever from the myriad other causes of febrile exanthems.
The diagnosis is also frequently overlooked in patients who do
not present with the typical rash or in whom a history of tick bite
cannot be elicited.

TABLE 1-44. DIFFERENTIAL DIAGNOSIS IN ROCKY MOUNTAIN SPOTTED FEVER

Meningococcemia
Rubeola
Enteroviral infections
Typhoid fever
Endemic murine typhus
Rickettsialpox
Colorado tick fever
Tularemia
Immune-complex vasculitis
Collagen vascular diseases
Thrombotic thrombocytopenic purpura
Idiopathic thrombocytopenic purpura

Treatment of the disease should be instituted as soon as the
diagnosis is suspected clinically. In addition to antibiotic therapy,
careful supportive intensive care is needed with aggressive intervention necessary to stabilize the most severely ill patients.

TABLE 1-45. TREATMENT OF ROCKY MOUNTAIN
SPOTTED FEVER

Chloramphenicol (100 mg/kg/day) or tetracycline (25 mg/kg/day)
  IV div q6h × 10 days; parenteral administration indicated for all
  but mildest cases of the disease
Attention to fluid management with replacement as needed of
  intravascular volume lost to 3rd spacing in order to restore
  circulation
Mechanical ventilation and PEEP may be needed to correct
  hypoxemia from noncardiogenic pulmonary edema
Replacement of platelets and clotting factors in cases with DIC and
  associated hemorrhage

SEPTIC SHOCK
No other problem is encountered as commonly in pediatric intensive care as sepsis. The diagnosis of sepsis in the child, particularly without an obvious source of infection, requires a high
degree of suspicion.

TABLE 1-46. CLINICAL DIAGNOSIS OF PRESUMED
SEPTICEMIA

Fever and chills, or hypothermia
Toxic appearance
Shock
DIC
Multiorgan failure
Documented source of infection
Host predisposition

TABLE 1-47. CLINICAL SYNDROMES COMMONLY ASSOCIATED WITH SEPSIS IN CHILDREN

Primary bacteremia	
Newborns	
Compromised host	Malignancy, immunodeficiency syndrome, immunosuppressive drug therapy
Normal children	Meningococcemia, pneumococcemia, *S. aureus* or β-hemolytic streptococcal septicemia
Secondary bacteremia	
Secondary to remote infection	Meningitis, osteomyelitis, septic arthritis, pneumonia, orbital cellulitis, wound infection, intestinal obstruction, pyelonephritis, burns, diarrhea
Secondary to operation or instrumentation	

Sepsis, if advanced, usually results in multiple organ system failure.

TABLE 1-48. EFFECTS OF SEPSIS ON ORGAN SYSTEMS

Hematologic	Granulocytosis, thrombocytopenia, DIC
Pulmonary	ARDS
Renal	Oliguria, acute renal insufficiency
Cardiac	Hypotension, myocardial depression (late)
Hepatic	Elevation of SGOT, SGPT, and bilirubin
Brain	Altered level of consciousness or confusion, especially with hypotension

Septic shock is encountered in a number of severe cases of sepsis, most commonly with gram-negative infections.

TABLE 1-49. INCIDENCE OF SHOCK WITH BACTEREMIA

Organism	Percentage with Shock
Gram-negative bacilli	42
S. aureus	29
S. pneumoniae	14

The cause and progression of unchecked septic shock is outlined in Table 1–50.

TABLE 1-50. PROGRESSION OF SEPTIC SHOCK

Early   Fever
Increased $\dot{V}O_2$
Increased cardiac output
Normal $A\bar{V}dO_2$
$\downarrow$
"Warm" shock
Vasodilatation
Decreased systemic vascular resistance
Redistribution of blood volume
Decreased preload
Increased cardiac output
Hypotension, wide pulse pressure
Oliguria, hypoxemia
$\downarrow$
Generalized capillary leak
Further decreased preload
Hypotension
Edema, ARDS
Multiple organ system dysfunction
$\downarrow$

Late   Oxygen extraction failure
Decreased VO_2 and $A\bar{V}dO_2$
Increased cardiac output
$\downarrow$
"Cold" shock
Vasoconstriction
Increased systemic vascular resistance
Release of myocardial depressant factor

(continued)

TABLE 1–50. (continued)

Poor coronary perfusion
Decreased cardiac output, increased $A\bar{V}dO_2$
Lactic acidosis
$\downarrow$
Death

TABLE 1–51. MANAGEMENT OF SEPTICEMIA IN CHILDREN

Attempt to identify source of infection	Careful physical examination, cultures, and radiographs as needed
Antibiotics	
Surgical exploration and/or drainage if indicated	
Monitor for the development of multi-organ system failure	Arterial blood pressure monitoring; accurate recording of fluid balance hourly; neurological checks hourly to assess level of consciousness; frequent ABG determinations and observation for signs of respiratory distress; determination of WBC, platelet count, HCT and liver and renal function tests may be desirable daily during acute phase of the illness

TABLE 1–52. INITIAL ANTIBIOTIC THERAPY FOR PRESUMED SEPTICEMIA OF UNKNOWN SOURCE

Neonatal	Ampicillin PLUS cefotaxime, ceftriaxone, moxalactam or gentamicin[a]
Pediatric	Cefotaxime, ceftriaxone, or moxalactam PLUS penicillin[a]
Immunocompromised host	Ticarcillin PLUS tobramycin PLUS nafcillin[a]

[a] See Tables 18–10 and 18–12 for dosages.

A general outline for treatment for septic shock should follow the familiar "A, B, C's" of cardiopulmonary resuscitation.

TABLE 1-53. TREATMENT OF SEPTIC SHOCK

Airway	Endotracheal intubation
Oxygenation	Mechanical ventilation with supplemental oxygen; PEEP as needed to correct hypoxemia if ARDS is present; goal is >99% arterial oxyhemoglobin saturation
Cardiac output	Transfusion of packed RBCs as needed to assure optimal red cell mass for adequate tissue oxygen delivery; optimize preload using fluid resuscitation with isotonic crystalloid solution or colloid (20 ml/kg over 20 min repeated as needed until circulation has stabilized or CVP >10 mm Hg or PCWP >12 mm Hg); correct acidosis (bicarbonate if pH <7.2, 0.3 × base deficit × wt in kg) or hypocalcemia, if present; inotropic support indicated if preload has been optimized and cardiac output is still insufficient to meet tissue oxygen demands; vasoactive agents as needed to maintain normal systemic vascular resistance.
Steroids	Methylprednisolone 30 mg/kg (maximum single dose 2 g) IV is beneficial if used early; repeat × 1 in 4–8 hr if patient remains unstable
Access and monitor- ing lines	IV Arterial line CVP or PCWP Urinary catheter NG tube (buffer gastric pH)

TETANUS

Tetanus is caused by the organism *Clostridium tetani*, which exists in both vegetative and sporulated forms. Spores may be introduced into a wound and may convert into the vegetative form producing a potent exotoxin, tetanospasmin, which affects the nervous system in several ways.

The incubation period for the development of tetanus is usually 3 days to 3 weeks. There are four forms of the disease with distinct presentations. Generalized tetanus is the most common. Cephalic tetanus is unusual and is seen following otitis media or injuries to the head and face. Neonatal tetanus usually presents in the first week of life after a contaminated delivery.

TABLE 1-54. CLINICAL MANIFESTATIONS OF TETANUS

Localized tetanus	Pain and continuous rigidity and spasm of muscles in proximity to site of injury
Generalized tetanus	Trismus, dysphagia, restlessness, irritability, headache, risus sardonicus, tonic contractions of somatic musculature, opisthotonus, tetanic seizures, spasm of laryngeal and respiratory muscles with airway obstruction, urinary retention, fever, hyperhydrosis, tachycardia, hypertension, cardiac arrhythmias
Cephalic tetanus	Dysfunction of cranial nerves III, IV, VII, IX, X, XI
Tetanus neonatorum	Difficulty sucking, excessive crying, dysphagia, opisthotonus, spasms

The diagnosis of tetanus is essentially a clinical diagnosis with a history of injury followed by the development of the symptoms described above. Laboratory findings are nonspecific in most cases.

Treatment focuses on removal of the source of toxin, neutralization of toxin, and supportive care until the toxin (which is fixed to neural tissue) can be metabolized. The average mortality of tetanus is 50% with even greater mortality for neonates. Recovery from tetanus does not confer immunity. Prevention is best accomplished by active immunization.

TABLE 1-55. TREATMENT OF TETANUS

Antitoxin	Tetanus immune globulin 3000–6000 U IM; begin tetanus toxoid active immunization
Antibiotics	Parenteral penicillin (200,000 U/kg/day) or tetracycline (30–40 mg/kg/day) × 10–14 days to eliminate vegetative forms of *C. tetani*
Surgical wound care	
Supportive measures	Decrease external stimuli such as noise and light
	Endotracheal intubation or tracheostomy as needed to protect against laryngospasm and aspiration
	Sedation
	Barbiturates, muscle relaxants, or neuromuscular blocking agents to decrease severity of muscle spasms
	Assure adequate ventilation using mechanical ventilator, if needed
	Treatment of sympathetic nervous system overactivity (extreme hypertension and tachycardia) cautiously with β and/or α adrenergic blockers
	Nutritional support

TOXIC SHOCK SYNDROME (TSS)

TSS is a recently recognized illness most commonly seen in young menstruating women, though it is occasionally present in other clinical settings.

TABLE 1-56. TSS

Onset of symptoms	
Menstrual cases	1–11 days after vaginal bleeding begins
Surgical wounds	2 days after surgery
Skin, subcutaneous soft tissue, wound, or osseous infection	1 day–8 wk
Postpartum and postabortion cases	1 day–8 wk

The syndrome is characterized by a constellation of findings.

TABLE 1-57. CLINICAL MANIFESTATIONS OF TSS

Signs	Symptoms
Rash	Myalgia
Desquamation	Vomiting
Fever	Dizziness
Hypotension	Sore throat
Pharyngitis	Headache
Strawberry tongue	Diarrhea
Conjunctivitis	Arthralgia
Vaginitis	Cough
Edema	
Confusion	
Agitation	
Somnolence	
Polyarthritis	

TABLE 1-58. CRITERIA FOR DIAGNOSIS OF TSS

Temperature $\geq$ 38.9C
Diffuse macular erythroderma or polymorphic maculopapular rash
Desquamation of palms or soles 1–2 wk after onset of illness
Hypotension: systolic BP $\leq$ 90 mm Hg (adults) or < 5th percentile by age (children < 16 yr), or orthostatic dizziness or syncope
Involvement of three or more of the following organ systems:
    GI (vomiting or diarrhea at onset of illness)
    Hepatic (total bilirubin, SGOT, or SGPT $\geq$ 2 × upper normal value)
    Hematologic (platelet count $\leq$ 100,000 mm^3)
    Mucous membrane (conjunctival, pharyngeal, or vaginal hyperemia)
    Muscular (severe myalgia or creatine phosphokinase $\geq$ 2 × upper normal value)
    Renal ($\geq$ 5 WBCs per high power field or BUN or creatinine $\geq$ 2 × upper normal value)
    CNS (disorientation or altered level of consciousness without focal neurologic signs when fever and hypotension absent)
    Metabolic (decreased total serum protein, albumin, calcium, and/or phosphorus)
Reasonable evidence for absence of other bacterial, viral, or rickettsial infection, drug reaction, or autoimmune disorder

TABLE 1-59. LABORATORY ABNORMALITIES IN TSS

Low serum calcium
Low serum phosphorus
Low total serum protein
Hypoalbuminemia
Leukocytosis with left shift
Anemia
Thrombocytopenia
Elevation of liver function tests (bilirubin, SGOT, SGPT,
  prothrombin time)
Elevation of renal function tests (BUN, Cr)
Pyuria
Elevation of serum creatine phosphokinase

TABLE 1-60. FACTORS ASSOCIATED WITH INCREASED RISK FOR TSS

1. Previous history of vaginal infection
2. Similar illness during a previous menstrual period
3. Use of tampons, particularly highly absorbent brands

Although the etiology is still unclear, there is a strong link between the isolation of *S. aureus* from vagina or cervix and the occurrence of the syndrome. This is usually in association with negative blood cultures, implicating a staphylococcal pyrogenic exotoxin as causative for the symptoms.

TABLE 1-61. TREATMENT OF TSS

Supportive intensive care	See Septic Shock (Table 1–53)
Antibiotics	Nafcillin 150 mg/kg/day IV div q6h
Discontinue tampon use	
Steroids (see Table 1-53)	

2

Neonatal Infection

SEPSIS, MENINGITIS AND PNEUMONIA

Serious bacterial infections occur in one to ten babies per 1000 live births. Despite the use of antibiotics and neonatal intensive care, mortality from these infections is as high as 30% and morbidity is significant in the survivors, particularly in those who had meningitis.

Newborns at high risk to infection can be identified by recognizing certain predisposing perinatal complications. Prematurity is the most common factor, increasing the incidence of sepsis fourfold. Prolonged rupture of the membranes for more than 24 hours prior to delivery, maternal chorioamnionitis, low socio-economic status, male gender, and low Apgar scores are all associated with a greater incidence of infection. Identification of infected newborns is difficult because the clinical signs and symptoms are nonspecific and often subtle. The signs seen in neonatal sepsis may also be seen in a variety of noninfectious diseases.

TABLE 2-1. SIGNS OF NEONATAL SEPSIS

Thermal instability	Fever, hypothermia
Respiratory distress	Tachypnea, grunting, apnea
Feeding disturbance	Gastric residuals, vomiting, poor feeding
CNS dysfunction	Lethargy, irritability, seizures

The laboratory results can help distinguish infections from other neonatal illnesses. The most useful test is the WBC count and differential. An absolute neutrophil count below $5000/mm^3$ or an immature–total neutrophil ratio above 0.15 in the first 24 hours of life strongly suggests infection. Demonstration of WBC and bacteria on a gram stain of the gastric aspirate indicates increased risk for infection.

Cultures of the blood and CSF should be obtained in all infants suspected of serious bacterial infection. In addition, surface and gastric aspirate cultures may be helpful in the first 4 to 6 hours of life. Most infants with sepsis will have positive blood cultures, although occasional infants will not be bacteremic at the time the culture is obtained. Thus, culture results must be interpreted in the context of the clinical picture. About one third of infants with sepsis will also have meningitis. Culturing the CSF in infants with suspected sepsis is important because 15% of infants with meningitis have negative blood cultures. Most with meningitis will have abnormal values of CSF protein, glucose, or WBC count. The diagnosis of pneumonia depends upon demonstrating a typical focal or diffuse pulmonary infiltrate on chest x-ray. Infants with pneumonia are less likely to have positive blood cultures, but cultures of deep tracheal secretions may identify the responsible organism.

Etiology

Most infections occurring within the first 5 days of life are acquired through vertical transmission from the mother. Organisms can spread transplacentally, as an ascending infection prior to birth or by direct contact as the infant passes through the birth canal. Ascending infection through ruptured membranes and then subsequent aspiration of infected amniotic fluid is thought to be the most common mechanism of early infection.

The majority of neonatal infections are caused by group B streptococci and *Escherichia coli*, but a number of other organisms also cause sepsis, meningitis, and pneumonia in the newborn.

TABLE 2-2. BACTERIAL ETIOLOGY OF SERIOUS NEONATAL INFECTION

Organism	Percentage
Group B streptococci	30
E. coli	30–40
Other gram-negative enterics	15–20
Haemophilus	
Klebsiella-Enterobacter	
Pseudomonas	
Other gram-positive cocci	10
Enterococcus	
Streptococcus pneumoniae	
Staphylococcus	
Listeria monocytogenes	5

Late onset infection (after 1 wk of age) has been frequently associated with group B streptococcus and *L. monocytogenes*. Although colonization with these organisms may occur during delivery, acquisition from an environmental source is more likely. Late onset disease is usually insidious compared to early onset disease and commonly includes meningitis.

Therapy

When neonatal sepsis is suspected, empiric antibiotic therapy is begun. Agents are chosen based on a knowledge of the sensitivities of the more frequent pathogenic organisms. Generally, a penicillin (usually ampicillin) is chosen to provide coverage against the gram-positive organisms (particularly *Listeria* and group D streptococci) and is coupled with a third generation cephalosporin (ceftriaxone, cefotaxime, or moxalactam) or an aminoglycoside for gram negative pathogens (see Table 18–10 for doses). Once the organism is identified, antibiotics can be adjusted to provide more specific coverage. If the onset of infection is after 3 to 5 days of life, methicillin should be added, particularly for pneumonia. Duration of therapy depends upon culture results and clinical course.

TABLE 2–3. MANAGEMENT OF SUSPECTED NEONATAL SEPSIS

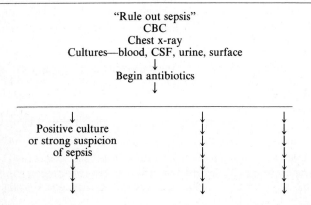

TABLE 2-3. (continued)

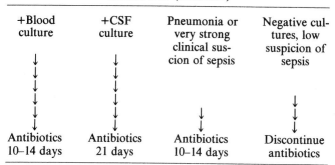

+Blood culture	+CSF culture	Pneumonia or very strong clinical suscion of sepsis	Negative cultures, low suspicion of sepsis
↓ ↓ ↓ ↓ ↓ ↓	↓ ↓ ↓ ↓ ↓ ↓	↓ ↓ ↓	↓ ↓ ↓
Antibiotics 10–14 days	Antibiotics 21 days	Antibiotics 10–14 days	Discontinue antibiotics

In addition to antibiotic therapy, careful supportive therapy is important in minimizing morbidity and mortality from neonatal infections. Thermal regulation, maintenance of proper fluid and electrolyte balance, and ventilatory assistance, if needed, are essential for optimal prognosis.

In an effort to further reduce morbidity and mortality, adjunct therapies have been recommended. Transfusion of whole blood or plasma has been used to improve perfusion and to provide complement and type-specific antibody thereby enhancing humoral and cellular immunity. Using a similar rationale, exchange transfusion has been used, with added proposed benefits of improving oxygen transport and "washing-out" bacteria and toxins. Evidence for the efficacy of these procedures remains largely anecdotal. Recognizing that many septic newborns are severely neutropenic, WBC transfusions have been utilized in this group; preliminary data suggest that survival is improved in infected newborns.

TORCH AND OTHER VIRAL INFECTIONS

Congenital infections occur in an estimated 7% of all live births. Recognition and management are necessary to minimize morbidity and mortality. The more common pathogens, *Toxoplasma*, rubella, cytomegalovirus (CMV) and herpes simplex virus (HSV)

are conveniently referred to as TORCH agents. These present
with similar clinical features making etiologic diagnosis a major
challenge in pediatric practice. Bacterial sepsis and syphilis may
also present with similar features and must be differentiated as
these require early therapeutic intervention. In addition, specific
therapy is available for herpes simplex (adenine arabinoside or
acyclovir; see Table 18-17) and for toxoplasmosis (see Table 2-6).
Diagnosis of rubella and herpes simplex is also important for
proper isolation of these cases.

TABLE 2-4. CHARACTERISTIC FINDINGS OF TORCH AGENT INFECTIONS

	Toxo-plasma	Rubella	CMV	Herpes
Microcephaly	+/−	+	++	+/−
Cerebral calcifications	++D	0	++PV	+/−
Hydrocephaly	++	0	+/−	+/−
Encephalitis	++	++	+/−	++
Hepatomegaly	++	++	++	++
Splenomegaly	++	++	++	++
Jaundice	++	+	++	++
Anemia	++	+	+	0
Thrombocytopenia	+	++	++	++
Petechiae/purpura	+	++	++	+
Vesicular rash	0	0	0	++
Macular rash	0	0	0	+
Cataracts	0	++	+/−	0
Chorioretinitis	++	++D	++F	+/−
Deafness	+	++	++	0
Congenital heart disease	0	++	+/−	0
Pneumonitis	+/−	++	+	+
Lymphadenopathy	+	++	+	0
Prematurity	+	+	++	+
IUGR	+	++	++	0
Osteochondritis/ bone lucencies	0	++	0	+/−

0 = not a feature; + = occasionally seen; ++ = prominent feature;
PV = periventricular; F = focal; D = diffuse.

An appropriate laboratory examination should be undertaken as soon as the clinical spectrum compatible with a TORCH agent infection is identified. In addition, a newborn with intrauterine growth retardation including height, weight, *and* head circumference measurements should also be evaluated.

TABLE 2–5. LABORATORY EXAMINATION OF TORCH AGENTS

Minimum Studies on Neonate

General: CBC, serum for IgM, serum to "hold"
    Toxoplasmosis: Acute and convalescent sera for Sabin-Feldman dye test, IHA or IgM-IFA; skull x-rays, CSF for pleocytosis and elevated protein
    Others: Bacterial sepsis: blood culture, CSF examination, bladder tap; syphilis: VDRL, x-rays of long bones
    Rubella: Acute and convalescent sera for HI; x-rays of long bones
    CMV: Urine for culture; skull x-rays
    Herpes simplex 1 and 2: Culture of CSF, vesicle (if present), or nasopharynx; Tzanck test of vesicle fluid

Summary of Specimens

Blood: Culture for bacteria, CBC, IgM, toxoplasmosis serology, rubella serology, VDRL, serum to "hold"
Urine: Culture for bacteria, culture for CMV
CSF: Culture for bacteria, culture for herpes simplex, cell count, protein, glucose, gram stain
X-ray: Long bones, skull series
Mother: Blood for VDRL, toxoplasma and rubella serology, serum to "hold," culture of cervix for group B streptococcus, herpes simplex, and CMV

Additional Studies When Organism Is Highly Suspected

Toxoplasmosis: CSF sediment (Wright's or Giemsa stain); culture of placenta and blood
Syphilis: Serum for FTA-abs or MHA-TP; convalescent serum for VDRL, FTA-abs or MHA-TP
Rubella: Culture of placenta, pharynx, urine, and stool
CMV: Culture of pharynx and liver biopsy; acute and convalescent serum for antibody (CF, FA, IHA, P, neutralization)
HSV: Acute and convalescent sera (CF or HA antibodies)

Toxoplasmosis

Congenital toxoplasmosis is due to transplacentally acquired fetal infection by *Toxoplasma gondii*. It occurs in approximately 1 in 1000 deliveries, and the majority of infants are asymptomatic at birth with sequelae recognized later in life. Fetal infection is seen in about 60% of primary maternal infection.

The diagnosis of congenital toxoplasmosis is usually entertained in an infant showing the "classical triad" of hydrocephalus, chorioretinitis, and intracranial calcifications. When clinically recognized in the neonate, the infection is usually severe, featuring prominent neurologic signs as well as evidence of generalized infection. Major sequelae include convulsions, mental retardation, and deafness.

TABLE 2–6. TREATMENT OF TOXOPLASMOSIS

Pyrimethamine (1 mg/kg/day PO div q12h) *PLUS*
Sulfadiazine (50–150 mg/kg/day PO div q6h) × 21 days
Possibly repeat 3–4 times in 1st yr of life
Folinic acid (calcium leucovorin) 5–10 mg/day
No isolation is required

Rubella

Rubella virus is transmitted across the placenta during the course of primary maternal infection. Intrauterine infection most commonly occurs in the first 8 weeks of pregnancy and decreases with advancing gestation. Eighty-five percent of infants infected during the first 8 weeks of gestation will have detectable defects, in contrast to 16% of infants infected near 20 weeks.

The most common malformations secondary to rubella are cardiac defects, diffuse "salt and pepper" retinopathy, cataracts, and deafness. Treatment is supportive and expectant with long-term follow-up to detect deafness and brain dysfunction.

CMV

CMV is the most common perinatally acquired infection. The newborn infant infected with CMV may present clinically in a variety of ways depending on whether there was early interference with organogenesis or infection of completely formed tissues late in pregnancy. The "typical" findings of congenital CMV are only seen in 5 to 10% of total cases. More subtle infections result in varying degrees of hearing loss. Diagnosis can be made on clinical, virologic, and serologic grounds.

It is becoming increasingly clear that the newborn infant is at risk to develop an acquired form of CMV infection from the transfusion of blood containing the virus.

TABLE 2–7. FEATURES OF TRANSFUSION-ACQUIRED CMV INFECTION

Infants at risk	Initially CMV-antibody negative
	> 50 ml total blood tranfused
	More than five separate blood donors
Manifestations	Pneumonia, hemolytic anemia, hepatitis, encephalitis
Prevention	Use only CMV-antibody negative blood
	Use of frozen deglycerolyzed blood, regardless of CMV antibody status

Herpes Simplex

HSV types I and II cause maternal herpes genitalis. Although HSV infection during pregnancy has been linked to congenital anomalies, abortion, and premature delivery, the major perinatal risk is neonatal disease following acquisition of the virus from the birth canal during delivery or by ascending infection following rupture of the membranes. The incidence of neonatal disease remains low, 0.2 to 0.5 per 1000 births. Heightened awareness of HSV infection has developed in recent years and the incidence of genital HSV infections has increased in certain segments of the adult population. The number of reported cases of neonatal disease has increased dramatically in recent years.

The risk of neonatal disease is probably greatest following vaginal delivery at the time of maternal primary HSV genital infection and may be as high as 40 to 50%. Vaginal delivery during episodes of recurrent disease, including times of asymptomatic shedding of virus, also places the neonate at significant risk with 70% of infected neonates being delivered to asymptomatic women. Cesarean delivery prior to rupture of the fetal membranes is recommended when genital lesions are present or a recent cervical culture for HSV has been positive. Rupture of the membranes for 6 hours increases the chance of ascending infection and lowers the preventive effect of cesarean delivery, although cesarean section at up to 24 hours following rupture of membranes is recommended by some. Nosocomial HSV infection in neonates has been documented with spread occurring indirectly from infected neonates or from infected nursery personnel. Isolation of infected neonates is required and has also been recommended for neonates at risk for disease. Rooming in and early discharge can be used to separate these neonates from the nursery environment.

Neonatal herpes infection usually presents as a rapidly progressive disease in the first or second week of life (average 6 days) with nonspecific signs of neonatal infection. Liver and adrenal gland involvement is common and CNS spread occurs in about half. Skin lesions are present in only 30% of patients with disease. Another group representing about one-third of the total cases, present with localized infection, particularly of the CNS with an average onset of 11 days but ranging up to 4 weeks.

Diagnosis of neonatal HSV is suggested by the clinical presentation and distinction from other infectious or noninfectious disorders will usually depend on isolation of the virus. Therefore, a high index of clinical suspicion must be maintained with particular attention to the prenatal history. Neonates at high risk for disease, such as those delivered vaginally in the presence of maternal infection or positive culture should be cultured and observed in the hospital for early signs of illness for 10 to 14 days. Those at lower risk should be discharged to the parents' care after careful instruction regarding signs of neonatal illness and plan for follow-up evaluation.

The prognosis has been grave for both forms of neonatal HSV infection with 80% mortality in disseminated disease and 48% in localized CNS disease. Survivors have commonly had severe neurologic sequelae. Early treatment with ara-A or acyclovir offers promise of improved outcome (see Table 18-17).

Other Viruses

The enterovirus group (Coxsackie virus, echo virus, and polio virus) is responsible for congenital and neonatal infections. No definitive evidence exists for transplacental transmission or ascending infection, and primary acquisition is thought to occur at the time of delivery. There is a distinct seasonal distribution in the United States, with a peak of infection from July through October. Clinical presentations depend on the specific virus and time in gestation.

TABLE 2-8. NEONATAL ENTEROVIRUS INFECTIONS

Features	Fever, poor feeding, diarrhea, lethargy, apnea, jaundice, myocarditis, meningitis, rash
Diagnosis	Culture nasopharynx, stool, CSF
Therapy	Supportive, isolation

The clinical differentiation of enteroviral and treatable bacterial disease is often difficult, but a summer to fall occurrence coupled with maternal symptoms of infection (fever, malaise, and diarrhea) plus evidence in the infant of aseptic meningitis, myocarditis, and/or diarrhea with fever should heighten suspicion of enteroviral illness.

Respiratory Syncytial Virus (RSV)

RSV infections are frequently acquired by infants in the first few weeks of life and may be associated with a high mortality rate, particularly if the infant is premature or has underlying lung or heart disease. Spread is by direct contact and droplet contamination. Nosocomial outbreaks have been reported in intensive care nurseries and most commonly occur during the winter and early spring months.

TABLE 2-9. NEONATAL RSV INFECTIONS

Features	Upper respiratory infection in winter or early spring
	Fever, apnea, dyspnea, pneumonia
Diagnosis	Culture RSV from respiratory tract secretions
Therapy	Supportive, respiratory isolation

COMMON FOCAL INFECTIONS

Conjunctivitis

The most frequently seen conjunctivitis in the newborn is due to chemical irritation from silver nitrate in the first 24 hours. Eye discharge beginning after 48 hours must be considered infectious. Because the clinical features and age of onset are similar, diagnosis of these infections is based on gram stains and cultures.

Ophthalmia neonatorum describes gonococcal conjunctivitis occurring within the first 3 weeks of life. The incidence has decreased from 24% in the early twentieth century, to less than 1% since the institution of silver nitrate prophylaxis.

TABLE 2-10. COMMON NEONATAL EYE INFECTIONS

Infecting Organism	Age of Onset	Clinical Features	Therapy
Chlamydia trachomatis	3–13 days	Unilateral or bilateral mild conjunctivitis, copious purulent discharge	Topical erythromycin, tetracycline, or 10% sodium sulfacetamide and oral erythromycin
Neisseria gonorrhoeae	2–5 days	Bilateral hyperemia and chemosis; copious thick white discharge	Penicillin G, IV (see Table 15–6) saline irrigation, strict isolation

TABLE 2-10. (continued)

Infecting Organism	Age of Onset	Clinical Features	Therapy
Staphylococcus aureus	2–5 days	Unilateral crusted purulent discharge	Topical sulfacetamide, neomycin, tetracycline or erythromycin methicillin IV for more serious infection (see Table 18-10 for dosages)

Omphalitis

Omphalitis is characterized by erythema, induration, and a serous or purulent discharge from the umbilical stump or periumbilical tissues. Microorganisms causing omphalitis are those normally present in the maternal birth canal, and include coagulase negative *Staphylococcus*, group A and B streptococci, diphtheroids, gram-negative enteric bacilli, and rarely *Clostridium tetani*.

Complications may include septicemia, septic umbilical arteritis, suppurative thrombophlebitis of umbilical or portal veins or the ductus venosus, peritonitis, scrotal or deep thigh abscess, liver abscess, endocarditis, pylephlebitis, subacute necrotizing funisitis, and portal vein thrombosis with resultant portal hypertension. Recommended initial therapy is intravenous methicillin plus gentamicin or ceftriaxone (see Table 18-10 for dosages).

Scalp Abscess

Fetal monitoring with internal scalp electrodes may result in a break in skin continuity with subsequent abscess formation. Treatment consists of local antiseptic care, incision, and drainage. If there is evidence of extension or systemic illness, parenteral antibiotics should be used based on microbiologic sensitivity.

NOSOCOMIAL INFECTION

Nosocomial infection in the newborn is defined as an infection
that was neither present nor incubating at birth, generally occurring 48 hours or more after birth. There is a considerable range in
the incidence from 0.6% in the normal newborn nursery to 15% in
some neonatal ICUs. The incidence has also changed within nurseries following changes in infection control measures. Decreased
rates have been attributed to increased nursing staff, increased
space per infant, convenient sinks and isolation facilities, i.e.,
overall improvement in staffing and environment.

TABLE 2–11. NOSOCOMIAL INFECTION ACCORDING TO BIRTH WEIGHT

Birthweight (g)	Utah (%)	Boston (%)
<1000	25/55 (45.4)	8/48 (18.4)
1000–1499	42/149 (28.1)	14/114 (13.0)
1500–1999	18/160 (11.2)	9/97 (9.3)
2000–2499	20/172 (11.6)	7/383 (1.8)
<2500	33/368 (8.0)	

Other major risk factors include length of hospitalization, surgery, supportive measures (e.g., endotracheal tubes, arterial catheters, hyperalimentation), immature host-defense mechanism,
and crowding.

There is general agreement that a large number of pathogenic
organisms may potentially cause nosocomial infection in newborns. However, a large percentage are due to one of the following: *S. aureus, E. coli, Klebsiella* sp., or *Pseudomonas aeruginosa*.
In many cases, the organisms colonize one or more surface sites
including wounds, burns, IV sites, or abrasions from tape application.

TABLE 2-12. COMMON ORGANISMS AND SITES OF NOSOCOMIAL INFECTION

	Surface (%)	Pneumonia (%)	Bacteremia (%)	Wound (%)	UTI (%)	Meningitis (%)
S. aureus	56	27	6	5	3	0
E. coli	21	30	16	11	8	12
Klebsiella	35	23	17	23	0	0
Pseudomonas	58	16	0	25	0	0
Others (multiple)	14	17	53	40	0	0

The spread of nosocomial infections in neonatal ICUs is largely due to contact with the hands of personnel caring for the colonized newborn or with contaminated equipment. There is a significant reservoir of gram-negative organisms (*E. coli, Pseudomonas,* and *Klebsiella*) constantly present in most nurseries, and efforts to reduce the spread have been directed toward strict handwashing and cleansing of equipment. In most nurseries today both gowning and handwashing (before and after every contact) routines are followed. Some nurseries have discontinued the requirement for gowning unless the infant is removed from the isolette.

3

Prevention

ACTIVE IMMUNIZATION

Routine Vaccination
The ultimate goal in medicine is not treatment but prevention of disease. Vaccine administration represents the most efficacious and cost effective measure for preventing infectious processes.

Success of this approach is best supported by eradication of smallpox and control of previously common severe infectious diseases such as polio, measles, diphtheria, and pertussis. There are presently 25 vaccines available in the United States (Table 3–1) and of these, eight should be routinely administered to all children prior to beginning school. These include diphtheria, tetanus toxoid, pertussis, trivalent oral polio, measles, mumps, rubella, and *H. influenzae*. The current recommendations from the Committee on Infectious Diseases, American Academy of Pediatrics (Report of the Committee on Infectious Diseases, 19th ed., 1982) for immunization in children are outlined in Table 3–2.

TABLE 3-1. VACCINES AVAILABLE FOR USE

Diphtheria	Smallpox	Typhoid
Tetanus	Pneumococcus	Tularemia
Pertussis	Rabies	Typhus
Polio	Meningococcus	Yellow fever
Measles	Cholera	Hepatitis B
Mumps	Plague	BCG
Rubella	Staphylococcus	Anthrax
H. influenzae	Arboviruses	Botulinum
Influenza		

TABLE 3-2. ROUTINE IMMUNIZATION SCHEDULE

Age	Vaccines
2 mo	DTP, oral polio
4 mo	DTP, oral polio
6 mo	DTP (oral polio is optional at 6 mo for areas at higher risk to imported cases, such as the southwestern U.S.)
12 mo	Tuberculin skin test (Monovac or Tine)
15 mo	MMR
18 mo	DTP, oral polio
24 mo	*H. influenzae*
5 yr	DTP, oral polio
15 yr	Adult Td
Adults	Td every 10 yr
All ages	Tetanus toxoid within 5 yr for "tetanus prone" wounds

Methods for providing these vaccines are certainly simple, essentially requiring only a concerned attitude on the part of parents and physicians. It is, therefore, unfortunate that over five million children in the United States are inadequately immunized against these eight infectious agents. Recent surveys of private pediatric practices have indicated that, even under optimal circumstances, 30 to 40% of preschool children were not appropriately vaccinated. In addition, screening for tuberculosis with intradermal skin testing should be accomplished at 12 months of age, then yearly in endemic areas. The general compliance with this recommended screening procedure is even lower.

Other Recommendations for Vaccine Use. If the immunization program for a young child is begun but not completed, the physician can simply continue where the program was interrupted. Original doses do not have to be repeated. There are, however, a few alterations. If the child is past the seventh birthday, pertussis vaccine should be eliminated and the adult form of diphtheria vaccine should be substituted. This diphtheria vaccine (Td) contains approximately 15% of material contained in childhood diphtheria. Otherwise, diphtheria-tetanus-pertussis (DTP) or adult tetanus diphtheria (Td) are given at 2-month intervals with measles-mumps-rubella (MMR) administered as soon as is practical.

Tetanus prophylaxis in wound management is simple if patients have received their primary immunization doses. Under these circumstances, tetanus toxoid, usually along with diphtheria, is given for a tetanus prone wound if the patient has not received tetanus toxoid within 5 years of the accident. If the individual has received two doses of tetanus toxoid during his or her lifetime, this is considered adequate and tetanus immune globulin need not be given. No doses or one dose of tetanus toxoid are both considered inadequate for protection and, under these circumstances for a tetanus prone wound, 500 U of tetanus immune globulin should be given along with tetanus toxoid, and the immunization procedure should be completed during long-term management with the next dose of DTP or Td given 4 weeks later.

The simultaneous administration of vaccines, particularly when "catching-up" on immunization programs, is a common practice. A great deal of clinical data now support the efficacy of vaccines administered on the same day if circumstances make this the only practical approach. The one drawback is that simultaneously administered vaccines are more likely to give local or systemic side effects and, if any reaction is severe, the clinician would not know which agent was responsible.

Other vaccines are generally administered only to individuals traveling to foreign countries where other infectious agents are endemic. Pertinent information for these travelers is available in the periodic publication of a supplement to *Morbidity and Mortality Weekly Report* entitled "Health Information for International Travel," which can be obtained from the Superintendent of Documents, U.S. Government Printing Office, Washington, D.C. 20402 or from state health departments.

Local side effects, such as erythema and induration with tenderness, are common after the administration of all vaccines, but particularly with pertussis. Reactions are self-limited and do not require specific therapy, although some physicians routinely administer aspirin or acetaminophen prior to offering immunizations. A nodule may appear at the injection site and persist for several weeks but this should not be considered a significant reaction. Rarely, systemic reactions occur and these necessitate the alteration of immunization programs.

**TABLE 3-3. CONTRAINDICATIONS TO
IMMUNIZATIONS**

Reaction to previous dose
  Neurologic
  Allergic
Live vaccines
  Immunodeficiency
  Malignancy
  Immunosuppressive therapy
  Immunoglobulin, plasma, or blood transfusion within 2 mo
  Pregnancy

If reactions occur with DTP injections, the physician can usually assume that the pertussis antigen is the causative agent and immunizations should then be completed with TD or Td. The only contraindication to tetanus and diphtheria toxoids is the history of a neurologic or a severe hypersensitivity reaction following a previous dose when pertussis had been excluded. When the causative agent cannot be determined, skin testing may be useful with tetanus and diphtheria toxoids to document immediate hypersensitivity. Tetanus toxoid should not be routinely given more frequently than every 10 years since with more frequent injections a percentage of recipients will develop major local reactions. These are essentially Arthus reactions, resulting from very high serum tetanus antitoxin levels.

Other Contraindications to Pertussis Vaccine. Hypersensitivity to vaccine components, presence of an evolving neurologic disorder, or a history of a severe reaction (usually within 48 hours) following a previous dose are definitive contraindications to the receipt of pertussis vaccine. Some authorities recommend discontinuing pertussis vaccine for other severe reactions.

TABLE 3-4. CONSIDER DISCONTINUATION OF PERTUSSIS VACCINE

Excessive somnolence of 3 hr duration
Persistent crying or screaming of 3 hr duration
Temperature more than 105F (40.5C)

Influenza Vaccine

Annual vaccination is recommended for all with medical problems that would result in more extensive infection once they developed influenza and for all individuals with increased exposure to potential outbreaks.

TABLE 3-5. INFLUENZA VACCINE

Chronic diseases	Immunosuppressive therapy
Pulmonary	Age > 65 yr
Cardiac	Hospital personnel
Renal	School teachers
Diabetes mellitus	
Metabolic disorders	
Anemia	
Malignancies	

The type of vaccine and dosage recommended for various age groups vary with the vaccine prepared each year. Therefore, the physician should consult the package insert or the state health department for specific information.

Field trials of influenza vaccines in the past have usually shown vaccine efficacy in the range of 70 to 80%. The greatest success is achieved when the antigenic drift of viral strains is anticipated so that the vaccines would include appropriate components. Vaccines now provide protection for both influenza A and influenza B. If an individual receives a vaccine each year, only one dose is needed. If vaccine was not given during a previous year, however, often two doses are required for adequate immunization.

Outbreaks of influenza occur between October and the end of February. Therefore, the vaccine should be administered before or during the month of October and discontinued by March 1. Often, an outbreak that occurs in December or January, is not documented until February when it receives national attention. This is too late to begin an immunization program since, historically, cases rarely appear after March 1. The best and most efficient system is for the primary care physician to maintain a list of patients who should receive vaccine and, during the month of September, notify these patients so that they may plan for a brief office appointment. The most important aspect in assuring success for vaccination practices is a compulsive and methodical attitude on the part of primary care physicians. The individual patient cannot be expected to remember this aspect of health care.

Pneumococcal Polysaccharide Vaccine

A 23-valent pneumococcal vaccine, replacing the previous 14-valent product, is currently licensed for use in the United States. This vaccine contains polysaccharide antigens for the following Danish types of *Streptococcus pneumoniae*: 1, 2, 3, 4, 5, 6B, 7F, 8, 9N, 9V, 10A, 11A, 12F, 14, 15B, 17F, 18C, 19A, 19F, 20, 22F, 23F, and 33F.

The serotypes chosen for inclusion in the material have been responsible for causing between 80 and 85% of invasive pneumococcal disease. This vaccine has been shown in field trials to be greater than 80% efficacious. The patients who may be expected to receive maximum benefit from this vaccine are similar to those included in influenza programs. In contrast, pneumococcal disease is not communicable. Therefore, hospital personnel and teachers are not considered at risk and would not be candidates for routine vaccination.

TABLE 3-6. CONSIDERATIONS FOR PNEUMOCOCCAL VACCINE

Splenectomy	Alcoholism
Congenital splenic aplasia	Cirrhosis
Sickle cell disease	Diabetes mellitus
Nephrosis	Congestive heart failure
Renal failure	IgA deficiency
Renal transplant	Down's syndrome
Chronic obstructive pulmonary disease	Complement deficiency
Cystic fibrosis	Immunosuppressive therapy
Chronic pulmonary disease	Severe neurologic disease
Malignancy	Aspiration syndromes
CSF leaks	The elderly (> 65 yr)

Infants less than 2 years of age do not demonstrate the same degree of antibody response achieved in healthy adults and, therefore, will not receive as much benefit from vaccine administration. However, even newborn infants respond with antibody production against at least some strains contained in the vaccine and would obtain some benefit from its administration. Neonates with asplenia might be considered for immunization. In such individuals, vaccine should be repeated at approximately 6 months of age and then again at 2 years to maximize protection.

The duration of protection is unknown, thereby leaving the question unanswered as to whether booster doses should be given. At present, no such recommendation is made except for immunizing the young infant. This is because adverse reactions were much more common among adults who received booster doses. The safety in pregnant women has not been established, so pregnancy remains a contraindication to its use. It is not presently recommended to administer this vaccine to older children or adults who previously received the 14-valent vaccine (licensed in 1977).

Several studies have supported the efficacy and safety of administering pneumococcal vaccine along with influenza vaccine. Because the persons receiving vaccines are in similar groups, both vaccines can be accomplished during the same office visit.

Hepatitis B Virus Vaccine

An inactivated (noninfective) vaccine for hepatitis B virus (HBV) is now available and recommended for recognized high risk groups. This is accomplished with three IM injections of 1 ml (20 μg/ml) with the second and third doses following the first by 1 and 6 months, respectively. For immunocompromised patients and those on hemodialysis, each dose is doubled (2 ml; 40 μg). For children under 10 years of age, one-half the adult dose is used. The only major disadvantage is high cost; no untoward side effects have been reported during a 3-year postvaccination observation period.

Serologic surveys have defined risk groups based on the prevalence of markers for HBV infection in various populations. Greatest risk is seen in homosexually active males and users of illicit injectable drugs who demonstrate essentially a 100% lifetime infection rate. HBV vaccine is of no benefit to acute or chronic virus carriers but should be given along with hepatitis B immune globulin to infants of HBV-antigen positive mothers.

TABLE 3-7. INACTIVATED HBV VACCINE

Preexposure vaccination
    Health care workers
    Hospital staff
    Clients and staff of institutions for the mentally retarded
    Hemodialysis patients
    Homosexually active males
    Illicit injectable drug users
    Recipients of certain blood products
    Household and sexual contacts of HBV carriers
    Special high risk populations
    Inmates of long-term correctional facilities
Postexposure vaccination
    Infants born to HBsAg-positive mothers
    Sexual and household contacts of acute HBV cases and health
      workers who receive needle sticks from HBsAg-positive patients

TABLE 3-8. HBV VACCINE FOR INFANTS OF HBsAg-POSITIVE MOTHERS

Birth	HB immune globulin 0.5 ml IM within 12 hr of birth
	HB vaccine 0.5 ml IM within 7 days of birth
1 mo	HB vaccine
6 mo	HB vaccine

PASSIVE IMMUNIZATION

Immunoglobulin

Passive immunization may be accomplished by administering immunoglobulin (previously called immune serum globulin) to individuals exposed to infectious hepatitis or those traveling into endemic regions of the world where probability of exposure is significant. There are currently four indications for the use of passive immunization.

TABLE 3-9. USES AND DOSES OF IM IMMUNOGLOBULIN

Hepatitis A	0.02 ml/kg (maximum 2 ml)
Hepatitis B	0.12 ml/kg
Hypogammaglobulinemia	0.66 ml/kg q3wk
Measles	0.25 ml/kg

Efficacy has been established in a number of clinical studies. This material is made from a pool of human donors, at least some of whom would have been exposed to the agent in question. The use of the human product is far superior to using animal sera because reactions to human immunoglobulin are rare. Immunoglobulin contains almost entirely IgG. Therefore, no protective effects from the small quantities or IgA or IgM would be anticipated. Moreover, the short half-life of just 5 days for the latter two immunoglobulins is too short to offer any beneficial effect. Intravenous human immunoglobulin preparations have been developed and examined in a number of clinical immunology centers for tolerance and efficacy and are now available. The dose is 200 mg/kg administered once a month. Although systemic reactions have been observed and occur much more frequently than the current IM preparations, this product seems to be much better tolerated by those hypogammaglobulinemic patients who have to receive large volumes of immunoglobulins. Currently, the cost is high, which must also be considered in planning a program of long-term management.

Hyperimmune Human Immunoglobulin

In addition to pooled human immunoglobulin, gammaglobulin prepared from selected hyperimmune donors is particularly useful as passive immunotherapy in modifying or preventing clinical illness from a number of infectious agents.

TABLE 3-10. HYPERIMMUNE HUMAN IMMUNOGLOBULIN

Immune Globulin	Manufacturer
Rh_o-D	Cutter Biological, Armour, Ortho Diagnostic, Parke-Davis
Tetanus	Cutter Biological, Savage, Hyland, Parke-Davis, Wyeth, Elkins-Sinn, Merck Sharp and Dohme, Hyland Therapeutics
Rabies	Cutter Biological
Varicella-zoster	Massachusetts Public Health
Mumps	Cutter Biological
Hepatitis B	Cutter Biological, Abbott, Merck Sharp and Dohme

The need for consultation concerning the indications for varicella-zoster hyperimmune globulin (VZIG) is more frequent than for any of the other globulin products. This is the result of both the ubiquitous nature of the virus and the large number of patients who benefit from its administration. The most common circumstance is a child with malignancy, usually leukemia, who is exposed to chickenpox. Table 3-11 outlines the guidelines for using VZIG. It is now more readily available through regional distribution centers around the country, which are listed in Table 3-12.

TABLE 3-11. GUIDELINES FOR THE USE OF VZIG

1. One of the following underlying illnesses or conditions
   a. Leukemia or lymphoma
   b. Congenital or acquired immunodeficiency
   c. Under immunosuppressive treatment
   d. Newborn of mother who had onset of chickenpox <5 days before delivery or within 48 hr after delivery
2. One of the following types of exposure to chickenpox or zoster patient(s):
   a. Household contact
   b. Playmate contact (>1 hr play indoors)

(*continued*)

TABLE 3-11. (continued)

c. Hospital contact (in same 2- to 4-bed room or adjacent beds in a large ward)

d. Newborn contact (newborn of mother who had onset of chickenpox <5 days before delivery or within 48 hr after delivery)

3. Negative or unknown prior history of chickenpox
4. Age of <15 yr, with administration to older patients on an individual basis
5. Time elapsed after exposure is such that VZIG can be administered within 96 hr

TABLE 3-12. DISTRIBUTION CENTERS FOR VZIG

Regional Center Service Area	24-hour Telephone Number
Massachusetts	Massachusetts Public Health Biologic Laboratories 375 South Street Jamaica Plain, MA 02130 (617) 522-3700
Maine	American Red Cross Blood Service Northwest Region 812 Huntington Avenue Boston, MA 02115 (617) 731-2130, ext 146
Connecticut	American Red Cross Blood Services Connecticut Region 209 Farmington Avenue Farmington, CT 06032 (203) 678-2700 (203) 677-4538 (night)
Vermont, New Hampshire	American Red Cross Blood Services 32 North Prospect Street Burlington, VT 05402 (802) 658-6400

TABLE 3-12. (continued)

Regional Center Service Area	24-hour Telephone Number
Rhode Island	Rhode Island Blood Center 551 North Main Street Providence, RI 02917 (401) 863–8366
New Jersey, New York	The Greater New York Blood Program 150 Amsterdam Avenue New York, NY 10023 (212) 570–3067 (day) (212) 570–3068 (night)
Delaware, Pennsylvania	American Red Cross Blood Services Penn-Jersey Region 23rd and Chestnut Street Philadelphia, PA 19103 (215) 299–4114

Maryland, Virginia, Washington
  DC, West Virginia
	American Red Cross Blood
	  Program
	Washington Region
	2025 E. Street, NW
	Washington, DC 20006
	(202) 728–6429

Alabama, Georgia, Mississippi,
  North Carolina, Puerto Rico,
  South Carolina
	American Red Cross Blood
	  Services
	Atlanta Region
	1925 Monroe Drive, NE
	Atlanta, GA 30324
	(404) 881–9800, ext 244
	(404) 881–6752 (night)

Florida	South Florida Blood Service PO Box 420100 Miami, FL 33142 (305) 326–8888
Indiana, Michigan, Ohio	American Red Cross Blood Service Southeastern Michigan Region 100 Mack Avenue PO Box 351 Detroit, MI 48232 (313) 833–4440

(continued)

TABLE 3-12. (continued)

Regional Center Service Area	24-hour Telephone Number
Iowa, Minnesota, Nebraska, North Dakota, Northern Illinois, Chicago, South Dakota, Wisconsin	The Blood Center of Southeastern Wisconsin 170 Wisconsin Avenue Milwaukee, WI 53233 (414) 933–5003
Arkansas, Kansas, Kentucky, Missouri, Southern Illinois, Tennessee, Nebraska	American Red Cross Blood Services Missouri-Illinois Region 4050 Lindell Boulevard St. Louis, MO 63108 (314) 658–2000
Louisiana, Oklahoma, Texas	Gulf Coast Regional Blood Center 1400 La Concha Houston, TX 77054 (713) 791–6250
Arizona, Colorado, New Mexico	United Blood Services PO Box 25445 Albuquerque, NM 87125 (505) 247–9831
Hawaii, Southern California	American Red Cross Blood Services Los Angeles-Orange Counties Region 1130 South Vermont Avenue Los Angeles, CA 90006 (213) 739–5620
Nevada, Utah, Wyoming, Northern California	American Red Cross Blood Services Central California Region 333 McKendrie Street San Jose, CA 95110 (408) 292–6242; (408) 292–1626 (night)
Alaska, Idaho, Montana, Oregon, Washington	Puget Sound Blood Center Terry at Madison Seattle, WA 98104 (206) 292–6525

TABLE 3-12. (continued)

Regional Center Service Area	24-hour Telephone Number
Canada	Canadian Red Cross 222 St. Patrick Toronto, Ontario (416) 596–3230
All other countries	Massachusetts Public Health Biologic Laboratories 375 South Street Jamaica Plain, MA 02130 (617) 522–3700

Hyperimmune Animal Immunoglobulin

In addition to human hyperimmune globulin preparations, antisera of animal origin are also available for clinical use. These products carry with them a high probability of serum reactions, particularly if the recipient has been exposed to similar animal products previously. Information for these and other products can be obtained through the Centers for Disease Control, telephone: (404) 329–3311 or 329–3644. Materials include: black widow spider equine antivenin, equine western equine encephalitis, botulism ABE polyvalent equine antitoxin, diphtheria equine antitoxin, polyvalent gas gangrene equine antitoxin, coral snake equine antivenin, and crotalid polyvalent antivenin.

PROPHYLACTIC ANTIBIOTICS

Rheumatic Fever

(Adapted from current American Heart Association recommendations)

Primary Prevention. Group A streptococcal infections of the upper respiratory tract are the most common precipitating causes of rheumatic fever. It follows, therefore, that appropriate treatment of streptococcal upper respiratory tract infections will prevent most attacks of acute rheumatic fever. Penicillin is the drug of choice except in patients allergic to this drug. Either IM or oral therapy is appropriate, but if oral therapy is used, a full 10-day course of treatment is necessary. The choice between IM and oral penicillin depends upon the physician's assessment of the patient's likely compliance with an oral regimen and risks of rheumatic fever in the population group being served.

Secondary Prevention. Rheumatic subjects who develop a streptococcal upper respiratory tract infection are at high risk of developing a recurrent attack of acute rheumatic fever. Asymptomatic, as well as symptomatic, infections may trigger a recurrence. Even in optimally treated symptomatic infections, prevention may fail. For these reasons prevention of recurrent rheumatic fever depends upon continuous prophylaxis rather than solely upon recognition and treatment of acute episodes of streptococcal pharyngitis. In general, continuous antibiotic prophylaxis is recommended for patients who have a well-documented history of rheumatic fever (including cases manifested solely by Sydenham's chorea) or for those who show definite evidence of rheumatic heart disease. Such prophylaxis should be initiated as soon as the diagnosis of active rheumatic fever or rheumatic heart disease is made. In the case of patients with acute rheumatic fever a full therapeutic course of penicillin should first be given to eradicate group A streptococci which may or may not be recoverable on throat culture.

The most effective protection from rheumatic recurrences is afforded by long term continuous antibiotic prophylaxis, perhaps for life. It is known, however, that the risk of recurrence declines with the interval since the most recent attack. Moreover, patients without rheumatic heart disease are at less risk of recurrence than those with cardiac involvement. Therefore, physicians may wish to make exceptions to maintaining prophylaxis indefinitely on an individual basis especially in older individuals. In making such decisions the physician must carefully weigh a number of factors including the patient's risk of acquiring a streptococcal infection, the anticipated recurrence rate per infection, and the consequences of recurrence. Adults with a high risk of exposure to streptococcal infection include parents of young children, school teachers, physicians, nurses and allied medical personnel, military recruits, and others living in crowded situations. Prophylaxis should be continued in patients with rheumatic heart disease even after prosthetic valve replacement, because these patients remain at risk to developing recurrences of rheumatic fever.

TABLE 3-13. CHOICES OF RHEUMATIC FEVER PREVENTION PROGRAMS

Benzathine penicillin G	1.2 million U IM monthly (> 60 lb); 600,000 U (< 60 lb)
Penicillin V	250 mg PO bid (> 60 lb); 125 mg (< 60 lb)
Sulfadiazine and penicillin V are equally effective, sulfisoxazole is probably also effective	1.0 g qd (> 60 lb); 0.5 g (< 60 lb)
For patients allergic to both penicillin and sulfonamides, erythromycin may be effective	

Bacterial Endocarditis Prophylaxis. Patients with evidence of rheumatic valvular heart disease also require additional short term antibiotic prophylaxis at the time of any procedures to prevent possible development of bacterial endocarditis. Because these patients have been on continual penicillin prophylaxis, viridans streptococci in the oral cavity are frequently resistant to penicillin. When certain dental or surgical procedures are undertaken these patients should be protected by administration of appropriate antibiotics in recommended doses (usually erythromycin see Table 3-17). Patients who have had rheumatic fever but who do not have evidence of rheumatic heart disease do not need endocarditis prophylaxis.

Bacterial Endocarditis

Bacterial endocarditis is one of the most serious forms of cardiac disease. Morbidity and mortality from endocarditis continue to be substantial despite advances in antimicrobial therapy and cardiovascular surgery.

TABLE 3-14. CARDIAC CONDITIONS FOR WHICH ENDOCARDITIS PROPHYLAXIS IS RECOMMENDED[a]

1. Prosthetic cardiac valves (including biosynthetic valves)
2. Most congenital cardiac malformations
3. Surgically constructed systemic pulmonary shunts
4. Rheumatic and other acquired valvular dysfunction
5. IHSS
6. Previous history of bacterial endocarditis
7. Mitral valve prolapse with insufficiency[b]

[a] This table lists common conditions but is not meant to be all inclusive.
[b] Definitive data to provide guidance in management of patients with mitral valve prolapse are particularly limited. It is clear that in general such patients are at low risk to development of endocarditis, but the risk-benefit ratio of prophylaxis in mitral valve prolapse is uncertain.

TABLE 3-15. CARDIAC CONDITIONS FOR WHICH ENDOCARDITIS PROPHYLAXIS IS NOT RECOMMENDED

1. Isolated secundum atrial septal defect
2. Patients in whom a VSD has closed spontaneously
3. Postoperative ASD, PDA, VSD patients in whom there is no residual shunt

Dental Procedures and Upper Respiratory Tract Surgical Procedures. Antibiotic prophylaxis is recommended with *all* dental procedures (including routine professional cleaning) likely to cause gingival bleeding. Because the spontaneous shedding of deciduous teeth or simple adjustment of orthodontic appliances do not present a significant risk of endocarditis, antibiotics are not necessary. Similarly, endotracheal intubation is not an indication for antibiotic prophylaxis unless associated with another procedure for which prophylaxis is recommended.

Because α-hemolytic (viridans) streptococci are most commonly implicated in endocarditis following dental procedures, prophylaxis should be specifically directed against these organisms. Certain upper respiratory tract procedures (e.g., tonsillectomy and/or adenoidectomy, bronchoscopy— especially with a rigid bronchoscope—and surgical procedures including biopsy involving respiratory mucosa) may also cause bacteremia with organisms having similar antibiotic susceptibilities to those producing bacteremia following dental procedures. Therefore, the same regimens are recommended. Endocarditis has not been reported in association with insertion of tympanostomy tubes. Studies to define the risk of bacteremia with this procedure are not available, however.

Table 3–17 contains suggested regimens of prophylaxis for dental procedures, surgical procedures, and instrumentation of the upper respiratory tract. In those patients at particularly high risk for endocarditis (e.g., those with prosthetic heart valves or surgically constructed systemic pulmonary shunts), we favor the use of parenteral prophylactic antibiotics.

TABLE 3-16. PROCEDURES FOR WHICH ENDOCARDITIS PROPHYLAXIS IS INDICATED

1. All dental procedures likely to induce gingival bleeding (not simple adjustment of orthodontic appliances or shedding of deciduous teeth)
2. Tonsillectomy and/or adenoidectomy
3. Surgical procedures or biopsy involving respiratory mucosa
4. Bronchoscopy, especially with a rigid bronchoscope[a]
5. Incision and drainage of infected tissue
6. Genitourinary and gastrointestinal procedures as listed in text

[a] The risk with flexible bronchoscopy is low, but the necessity for prophylaxis is not yet defined.

TABLE 3-17. SUMMARY OF RECOMMENDED ANTIBIOTIC REGIMENS FOR DENTAL-RESPIRATORY TRACT PROCEDURES

Standard regimen	For dental procedures that cause gingival bleeding and oral/respiratory tract surgery	Penicillin V 2.0 g PO 1 hr before, then 1.0 g 6 hr later. For patients unable to take oral medications, 2 million U of aqueous penicillin G IV or IM 30–60 min before a procedure and 1 million U 6 hr later may be substituted
Special regimen	Parenteral regimen for use when maximal protection desired; e.g., for patients with prosthetic valves	Ampicillin 1.0–2.0 g IM or IV *PLUS* gentamicin 1.5 mg/kg IM or IV, ½ hr before procedure, followed by 1.0 g oral penicillin V 6 hr later. Alternatively the parenteral regimen may be repeated once 8 hr later
	Oral regimen for penicillin-allergic patients	Erythromycin 1.0 g PO 1 hr before, then 500 mg 6 hr later
	Rheumatic fever patients who have been on penicillin prophylaxis	Erythromycin as above
	Parenteral regimen for penicillin-allergic patients	Vancomycin 1.0 g IV *slowly* over 1 hr, starting 1 hr before. No repeat dose is necessary

Note: Pediatric doses: ampicillin 50 mg/kg dose; erythromycin 20 mg/kg for 1st dose, then 10 mg/kg; gentamicin 2.0 mg/kg dose; penicillin V full adult dose if > 60 lb, ½ adult dose if < 60 lb; aqueous penicillin G 50,000 U/kg (25,000 U/kg for follow-up); vancomycin 20 mg/kg dose. The intervals between doses are the same as for adults. Total doses should not exceed adult doses.

(Adapted from current American Heart Association recommendations.)

GU Tract, GI Tract Surgery and Instrumentation. Bacteremia often accompanies surgery or instrumentation of the GU or GI tract, and endocarditis may ensue. Data are inadequate to support specific recommendations to cover the entire range of invasive diagnostic and therapeutic procedures. Based upon the limited data available, the committee recommends prophylaxis for the following: cystoscopy, prostatic surgery, urethral catheterization (especially in the presence of infection), urinary tract surgery, vaginal hysterectomy, gall bladder surgery, colonic surgery, esophageal dilatation, sclerotherapy of esophageal varices, colonoscopy, upper GI endoscopy with biopsy, or proctosigmoidoscopic biopsy. Thus, patients at risk for bacterial endocarditis undergoing such procedures should receive prophylactic antibiotics as outlined below.

Bacteremia less often accompanies other GU and GI tract procedures, and endocarditis has developed subsequent to those procedures rarely, if ever. These include percutaneous liver biopsy, upper GI endoscopy or proctosigmoidoscopy without biopsy, barium enema, uncomplicated vaginal delivery, and brief ("in and out") bladder catheterization with sterile urine. If infection is not suspected, the following gynecologic procedures do not routinely require prophylaxis: uterine dilatation and curettage, cesarean section, therapeutic abortion, sterilization procedures (IUD insertion or removal remains a controversial issue and in general this method of birth control is not recommended for women with significant heart disease).

Because patients with prosthetic heart valves and those with surgically constructed systemic pulmonary shunts appear to be at especially high risk for infective endocarditis, it may be prudent to administer prophylactic antibiotics for these low risk procedures.

Enterococci (e.g, *Streptococcus faecalis*) are most frequently responsible for endocarditis following GU and GI tract surgery or instrumentation. Although gram-negative bacillary bacteremia may follow such procedures, these organisms are only rarely responsible for endocarditis. Thus, antibiotic prophylaxis to prevent endocarditis following these procedures should be directed primarily against enterococci.

<h3 style="text-align:center">TABLE 3-18. SUMMARY OF RECOMMENDED REGIMENS FOR GASTROINTESTINAL/GENITOURINARY PROCEDURES</h3>

Standard regimen	For genitourinary/ gastrointestinal trace procedures listed in the text	Ampicillin 2.0 g. IM or IV *PLUS* gentamicin 1.5 mg/kg IM or IV, given ½–1 hr before procedure. One follow-up dose may be given 8 hr later
Special regimen	Oral regimen for minor or repetitive procedure in low-risk patients	Amoxicillin 3.0 g PO 1 hr before procedure and 1.5 g 6 hr later
	Penicillin-allergic patients	Vancomycin 1.0 g IV *slowly* over 1 hr, *PLUS* gentamicin 1.5 mg/kg IM or IV given 1 hr before procedure. May be repeated once 8–12 hr later

Note: Pediatric doses: ampicillin 50 mg/kg/dose; gentamicin 2.0 mg/kg/dose; amoxicillin 50 mg/kg/dose; vancomycin 20 mg/kg/dose. The intervals between doses are the same as for adults. Total doses should not exceed adult doses.

(*Adapted from current American Heart Association recommendations.*)

Cardiac Surgery. Patients undergoing open heart surgery, especially with placement of prosthetic heart valves or prosthetic intravascular or intracardiac materials are at risk for bacterial endocarditis. Because the incidence of morbidity and mortality of endocarditis in such patients is high, maximum preventive efforts including prophylactic antibiotics are recommended.

Endocarditis associated with open heart surgery is most often due to *Staphylococcus aureus*, coagulase-negative staphylococci, or diphtheroids. Streptococci, gram-negative bacteria, and fungi are less common. No single antibiotic regimen is effective against all of these organisms. *Furthermore, prolonged use of broad spectrum antibiotics may predispose to superinfection with unusual or resistant microorganisms.*

Therefore, prophylaxis at the time of cardiac surgery should be directed primarily against staphylococci and should be of short duration. Penicillinase-resistant penicillins or "first-generation" cephalosporins are most often selected, although the choice of antibiotic should be influenced by each hospital's antibiotic susceptibility data. For example, high prevalence of infection by methicillin-resistant staphylococci in a particular institution should prompt consideration of vancomycin for preoperative prophylaxis. Prophylaxis should be started immediately before the operative procedure and continued for no more than 2 days postoperatively to minimize emergence of resistant microorganisms. The effects of cardiopulmonary bypass and compromised postoperative renal function on serum antibiotic levels should be considered and doses timed appropriately before and during the procedure.

Additional Notes. In susceptible patients, prophylaxis to prevent endocarditis is also indicated for surgical procedures on any infected or contaminated tissues including incision and drainage of abscesses. In these circumstances, regimens should be individualized but in most instances should include antibiotics effective against *S. aureus.*

Antibiotic prophylaxis for the surgical and dental procedures indicated above should also be given to patients with a documented previous episode of bacterial endocarditis, even in the absence of clinically detectable heart disease.

Patients with indwelling transvenous cardiac pacemakers appear to present a low risk of endocarditis; when such cases occur they are predominantly due to staphylococci. Dentists and physicians however, may choose to employ prophylactic antibiotics when dental and surgical procedures are performed in these patients. The same recommendations apply to renal dialysis patients with arteriovenous shunt appliances. Endocarditis prophylaxis also deserves consideration in patients with ventriculoatrial shunts for hydrocephalus, because there are documented cases of bacterial endocarditis in these patients.

Prophylactic antibiotics are *not* required in diagnostic cardiac catheterization angiography because with adequate aseptic techniques the occurrence of endocarditis following these procedures is extremely low.

Tuberculosis

Isoniazid (INH) prophylaxis at a dose of 10 mg/kg/day (maximum 300 mg) is recommended for children during specified clinical circumstances, which are associated with an increased incidence of subsequent active tuberculosis. The risk for a tuberculin reactor varies by age, sex, and race with the greatest being 10% in the young infant. The incidence is reduced by 70% with INH prophylaxis. Risk following household exposure to tuberculosis is 2 to 5% whereas the incidence of reactivation in an immunosuppressed individual is 15%.

TABLE 3-19. CHILDREN WHO SHOULD RECEIVE INH PROPHYLAXIS

	Duration of Treatment
Asymptomatic skin test reactor (≥ 10 mm) with a normal chest x-ray	1 yr
Skin test negative household contact of an active case	3 mo (then repeat skin test)
Previously skin test positive children who are immune suppressed (malignancy, corticosteroid, or immunosuppressive therapy)	For the duration of immune suppression

Meningococcal Disease

The secondary attack rate for household contacts of meningococcal meningitis or meningococcemia is 1/250 (0.4%). Rifampin prophylaxis at a dose of 20 mg/kg/day (maximum 600 mg) for 4 days effectively eliminates this risk. One-half this dose (10 mg/kg/day) may be used in neonates. Pregnancy is a contraindication to rifampin, but ceftriaxone, 125 mg IM as a single dose may be substituted. Soft contact lenses should be removed as rifampin causes permanent staining. Prophylaxis is also recommended for other groups that have had intimate contact with these patients.

TABLE 3-20. RIFAMPIN PROPHYLAXIS FOR MENINGOCOCCAL DISEASE

All household contacts
Nursery or daycare center contacts
Hospital personnel and individuals who had intimate exposure to
  oral secretions of index case

Haemophilus influenzae

The risk to household contacts of a child with invasive *H. influenzae* disease is 600 times higher than that in the general population and is age-dependent; the secondary attack rate for young infants less than 1 year is 6%, 1 to 4 years of age, 2.1%, and 4 to 6 years, 0.5%. The risk to contacts in day care centers has not been fully determined but appears to be great enough to warrant prophylaxis for children attending these centers and for adult personnel once there have been two cases of *H. influenzae* systemic disease. Rifampin prophylaxis for culture positive individuals has been shown to reduce the oropharyngeal carriage of *H. influenzae* by 97%.

Rifampin should be given at a dose of 20 mg/kg/day (maxi-

mum 600 mg) for 4 days. Pregnancy is a contraindication to prophylaxis and soft contact lenses should be removed during the
treatment period.

TABLE 3–21. RIFAMPIN PROPHYLAXIS FOR *H. INFLUENZAE* DISEASE

All household contacts, if the household contains a child < 4 yr
of age
Contacts in a day-care center (children and adults) following the
second case of invasive *H. influenzae* disease within 60 days
The last 4 days of hospitalization for the index case

Gonorrhea

Sexual contacts of documented gonococcal carriers are at significant risk to developing disease. Therefore, all such contacts,
whether adults, adolescents, or children should receive prophylaxis. Treatment regimens are essentially identical to those for
uncomplicated culture positive gonococcal infection (see Chap.
15).

TABLE 3–22. PROPHYLAXIS FOR GONOCOCCAL INFECTION

Amoxicillin	PO 50 mg/kg (maximum 3.0 g) as single dose *PLUS* probenecid PO 25 mg/kg (maximum 1.0 g)
	OR
Procaine penicillin G	IM 100,000 U/kg (maximum 4.8 million U) *PLUS* probenecid PO 25 mg/kg (maximum 1.0 g)
Penicillin-allergic individuals	Spectinomycin IM 40 mg/kg (maximum 2.0 g) single dose. Over 8 yr: tetracycline PO 25 mg/kg/day (maximum 2.0 g) div qid × 5 days

Syphilis
Because serologic conversion is delayed by 1 month following exposure to primary or secondary syphilis, contacts of such active cases should receive prophylactic antibiotics.

TABLE 3-23. PROPHYLAXIS FOR SYPHILIS

Benzathine penicillin G IM 50,000 U/kg (maximum 2.4 million U)
Allergy to penicillin
   Tetracycline PO 25 mg/kg/day (maximum 2.0 g) div qid × 15 days
   Erythromycin PO 50 mg/kg/day (maximum 2.0 g) div qid × 15 days

Pertussis
Prophylactic erythromycin is effective in preventing symptomatic disease as well as eradicating colonization in contacts of pertussis cases. Although immunization affords protection in 70 to 80% of recipients, prophylaxis should be offered to immunized as well as unimmunized family, daycare center, or hospital contacts during outbreaks of pertussis. Erythromycin is given PO 50 mg/kg/day (maximum 1.5 g) divided tid for 14 days.

Otitis Media
Although the usefulness of prophylactic antibiotics for the "otitis media prone" patient is controversial, this approach has become common practice. Adequate data for selecting appropriate patients and establishing duration of therapy do not yet exist. Published studies using various criteria, however, have supported efficacy. Table 3-24 summarizes previous guidelines for employing prophylactic antibiotics.

TABLE 3-24. PROPHYLAXIS FOR THE OTITIS MEDIA PRONE CHILD

Candidates for therapy
   2 episodes of otitis media in the 1st yr of life
   3 episodes within 6 mo at any age

(continued)

TABLE 3-24. (continued)

Duration of prophylaxis (any of the following)
   3 mo after an acute episode
   The duration of an episode of upper respiratory infection
   The winter months (usually November–April)
Antibiotic regimen (any of the following)
   Sulfisoxazole 75 mg/kg div bid
   TMP-SMX 4 mg TMP/20 mg SMX/kg single daily dose
   Ampicillin 125 mg < 2 yr of age; 250 mg > 2 yr of age; single
    daily dose

Urinary Tract Infections

Antibiotic suppressive therapy is occasionally necessary for children with anatomic defects of the urinary tract or with chronic indwelling urinary catheters. Every effort should first be made to correct such defects or to substitute periodic in-and-out catheterization.

A number of agents have been shown to be efficacious in preventing bacteriuria in girls who have had recurrent symptomatic UTIs. A search should first be made for correctable anatomic defects (see Chap. 10).

**TABLE 3-25. SUPPRESSIVE AND PROPHYLACTIC
THERAPY OF UTIs**

Suppression—single daily dose
   Nitrofurantoin PO 2 mg/kg
Prophylaxis—single daily dose
   TMP-SMX PO
     < 13 years 20 mg/100 mg
     > 13 years 40 mg/200 mg
   Nitrofurantoin PO 2 mg/kg

Common Outpatient Infections

Most infections can be managed on an outpatient basis and these comprise, by most estimates, 60 to 80% of unscheduled pediatric office or emergency room visits. Approximately 90% of febrile episodes in children are caused by viruses rather than bacteria and are usually accompanied by upper respiratory signs and symptoms. Reassurance and medication for fever or congestion are the only interventions warranted. Distinguishing more severe infectious processes remains the most important aspect of outpatient evaluation.

ABSCESSES (CUTANEOUS)

Organisms most frequently recovered from skin and soft tissue abscesses are *Staphylococcus aureus* and group A *β*-hemolytic streptococci. Among these infections, cutaneous abscesses should be distinguished from impetigo, cellulitis, and wound infections where treatment is somewhat different. All abscesses should be incised and drained. When there is a question as to whether a lesion is fluctuant, an 18-gauge needle and syringe can be used to aspirate material or probe the abscess. An incision can then be made and a wick placed to assure continued drainage. This is all that is necessary for *S. aureus* and most other organisms. Group A streptococci require penicillin or an appropriate alternative oral antibiotic. Bacteremia from cutaneous abscesses is extremely rare but should be considered with extensive involvement, high fever, or in the immunocompromised host.

TABLE 4-1. ORGANISMS RECOVERED FROM CUTANEOUS ABSCESSES IN CHILDREN

Aerobes (50%)
  S. aureus (25%)
  Group A *β*-hemolytic streptococci; *α*- and nonhemolytic
    streptococci
  Enterobacter
  E. coli
Anaerobes (25%)
  Bacteroides melaninogenicus
  Bacteroides fragilis
  Fusobacterium
Mixed aerobes and anaerobes (25%)

Abscesses in the perirectal region are almost always associated with anaerobic bacteria. As with other cutaneous abscesses, incision with drainage is the most important aspect of therapy. In contrast to infection in other anatomic areas, simple drainage may be inadequate. Fistulae must be identified, opened, and excised. Perirectal abscesses therefore require surgical consultation.

TABLE 4-2. ORGANISMS RECOVERED FROM PERIRECTAL ABSCESSES IN CHILDREN

Anaerobes (85%)
S. aureus (35%)
E. coli (20%)
Streptococci (10%)
Other aerobes (10%)

TABLE 4-3. TREATMENT OF CUTANEOUS ABSCESSES

Incision and drainage	
Antibiotics	Nafcillin + moxalactam (or as directed by gram stain and culture)
Only for	Extensive involvement, systemic symptoms, compromised host

ADENITIS

Adenitis should be distinguished from adenopathy (see Chap. 12) although considerable clinical overlap exists. Adenitis is usually painful, hot, and occurs more frequently (75%) in the 1- to 4-year-old age group. Untreated, these nodes will suppurate and occasionally progress to cellulitis and bacteremia. When there is no primary focus such as pharyngitis or tonsillitis, fever and other systemic symptoms imply such progression. Pitting edema strongly suggests the presence of a suppurative node that requires drainage. Cervical adenitis with minimal tenderness or persistence following 10 days of antimicrobial therapy increases the likelihood of atypical mycobacterial and *Mycobacterium tuberculosis* infection. This should be evaluated by intradermal testing with intermediate PPD (5 tuberculin units). Adenitis in all locations is caused most commonly by either *S. aureus* or group A streptococci and therapy is directed against these two pathogens.

TABLE 4–4. BACTERIAL ETIOLOGY OF ADENITIS

All locations	*S. aureus* 40–50%
	Group A streptococci 30–40%
Other organisms by location	
Cervical	Atypical mycobacteria
	M. tuberculosis
	Gram-negative enterics
	H. influenzae
	Anaerobes
	Actinomyces israelii
	Tularemia
Preauricular	Tularemia
Occipital	Tinea capitis
Axillary	Cat scratch disease
	Sporotrichosis
Inguinal	Anaerobes
	Gram-negative enterics
	Plague
Generalized	Infectious mononucleosis
	Toxoplasmosis
	CMV
	Other viruses
	Kawasaki disease
	Syphilis
	Hepatitis
	Brucellosis
	Sarcoidosis

TABLE 4–5. TREATMENT OF ADENITIS

Prescribe any of the following:
  Dicloxacillin or cloxacillin
  Erythromycin
  Cephalexin or cephradine
Each is given 50 mg/kg/day PO × 10 days
Incision and drainage when fluctuant

ANIMAL AND HUMAN BITES

Animal bites account for 1% of emergency room visits with 90% caused by dogs, 10% by cats, and 1% by rodents (rabbits, squirrels, hamsters, and gerbils). Approximately 90% are pets owned by the family or neighbors which suggests that better education of children (and parents) might reduce these all too common injuries. Human bites require similar management and are therefore included in this discussion.

A major focus of treatment concerns prevention of wound infection. Human bites most commonly become infected (greater than 50%), followed by cats (30%), whereas dog and rodent bites are associated with a 5% incidence of cellulitis or abscess formation. Such infection is usually clinically apparent within 24 hours after the injury. The much greater frequency of dogs being the offending animal accounts for greater clinical experience with these wounds. Upper extremity injuries become infected more commonly than those to the face, scalp or lower extremities. This is because debridement and irrigation of the compartments of the hand are more difficult. In contrast to animal attacks, human inflicted bites are not associated with infection caused by *Pasteurella multocida*.

TABLE 4-6. ORGANISMS RECOVERED FROM INFECTED ANIMAL BITES

P. multocida
S. aureus
Streptococcus sp.
Anaerobic bacteria

Gram stains or cultures immediately following the injury are not predictive of organisms subsequently associated with infection. Therefore, these laboratory studies should only be obtained once cellulitis or abscess formation occurs.

Every effort should be made primarily to close lacerations, both for cosmetic reasons and to reduce local bacterial colonization.

Large wounds, those associated with extensive tissue destruction, or ones requiring optimal cosmetic repair may best be managed under general anesthesia in the operating room.

TABLE 4-7. TREATMENT OF ANIMAL AND HUMAN BITES

Cleansing and debridement
Extensive wound irrigation
Suturing for closure
Antibiotics: penicillin + dicloxacillin
Tetanus prophylaxis when indicated
Rabies prophylaxis when indicated
Reexamine in 24 hr

BACTEREMIA

Reported studies have demonstrated a 4% incidence of bacteremia in febrile infants who do not appear toxic. The most common predisposing infections are otitis media and pneumonia. The majority of patients, however, have no obvious focus. Ninety percent of positive cultures yield pneumococcus or *Haemophilus influenzae*. Unique are children with sickle cell disease who exhibit a high incidence of pneumococcal bacteremia. These children, when febrile, require close observation.

TABLE 4-8. BACTEREMIA IN INFANTS

S. pneumonia (65%)
H. influenzae (25%)
N. meningitidis
Salmonella sp.
S. aureus

Febrile infants less than 2 months of age should usually be hospitalized and evaluated for sepsis. This includes blood culture, lumbar puncture, and urine for culture obtained by bladder tap or catheterization. Older infants are managed on an individual basis with decision for hospitalization based on physical assessment rather than any laboratory parameters. The decision to obtain a blood culture should usually be accompanied by one for observation in the hospital setting.

If bacteremia is documented from an outpatient culture, the patient should be reexamined. If improved but showing no focus of infection, amoxicillin 40 to 50 mg/kg/day PO divided tid × 10 days should be given. Specific infections should be treated as indicated. Those still febrile without a focus should be hospitalized for a sepsis workup.

CELLULITIS

Infection of the skin and subcutaneous tissue is most commonly the result of local trauma or the extension of an underlying abscess. Periorbital cellulitis more likely follows conjunctival colonization with *H. influenzae* whereas orbital cellulitis is a consequence of ethmoid sinusitis with penetration into the retrobulbar space. Buccal cellulitis is frequently associated with ipsilateral otitis media.

There are some features that help differentiate more likely etiologic agents. These should be used as guides to therapy.

TABLE 4-9. CELLULITIS: CLINICAL FEATURES ASSOCIATED WITH SPECIFIC BACTERIA

Clinical Feature	Organism
Neonate	
Facial	Group B streptococci
Funicitis (periumbilical)	Group A streptococci
Predisposing trauma	*S. aureus*
	Group A streptococci
Foot	*Pseudomonas* sp.
Burn	Group A streptococci
Chickenpox	Group A streptococci
	(continued)

TABLE 4–9. (continued)

Clinical Feature	Organism
Infant	
Facial, periorbital	*H. influenzae*
Violaceous hue (usually facial)	*H. influenzae*
	S. pneumoniae
Ascending lymphangitis	Group A streptococci
Erysipelas (distinct borders)	Group A streptococci

Selection of antibiotics is guided by an understanding of pathogens most likely to cause cellulitis. Any abscess should first be incised and drained. In most cases, a penicillinase-resistant penicillin is used to cover group A streptococci and staphylococci. When *H. influenzae* is a likely agent, such as with facial cellulitis, a third generation cephalosporin is most appropriate. Blood and an aspirate of the advancing margin of the cellulitis should be cultured.

TABLE 4–10. TREATMENT OF CELLULITIS

Neonate	Methicillin + Ceftriaxone
	Cefotaxime or moxalactam
1 mo–5 yr	
	Ceftriaxone
	Cefotaxime
	Moxalactam or chloramphenicol
Predisposing trauma	Nafcillin
Ascending lymphangitis	Penicillin

CONJUNCTIVITIS

Causes of conjunctivitis are largely age dependent and include sensitivity to environmental agents (allergic conjunctivitis) as well as viral and bacterial pathogens. Microscopic examination of exudate with gram stain and Giemsa stain for *Chlamydia trachomatis* when appropriate will help differentiate the varied etiologies. Cultures should be obtained prior to treatment.

TABLE 4-11. ETIOLOGY AND TREATMENT OF CONJUNCTIVITIS

Age	Etiology	Treatment
< 3 days	Silver nitrate	None
3 days–3 wk	*N. gonorrhoeae*	Penicillin
3 wk–16 wk	*C. trachomatis*	Sulfonamide eye drops *PLUS* erythromycin PO × 14 days
> 12 wk	*H. aegyptius* ("pink eye")	Sulfonamide eye drops × 5-10 days
	S. aureus	Topical bacitracin
	H. influenzae	Sulfonamide eye drops
	S. pneumoniae	Sulfonamide eye drops
	Moraxella lacunata	Sulfonamide eye drops
	Streptococci	Sulfonamide eye drops
	Adenoviruses	Cold soaks
	Enterovirus 70	Cold soaks
	Herpes simplex	Vidarabine ointment or trifluridine eye drops

DERMATOPHYTOSES AND CANDIDIASIS

Dermatophytes have the unique ability to colonize skin, hair, and nails but almost never invade deeper tissues. Diagnosis is made clinically by noting characteristic patterns such as a ring with central clearing or kerion formation. Confirmation is best achieved with a KOH preparation. Wood light examination will demonstrate the characteristic apple green fluorescence of *Microsporum* and some other organisms. Currently, 37 species of dermatophytes have been identified. It is more practical to approach diagnosis and selection of antifungal agents according to clinical presentation. Cultures are most useful for infections that do not respond to initial therapy.

TABLE 4-12. TREATMENT OF DERMATOPHYTOSES

Clinical Disease	Therapy
Tinea capitis	
Kerion	Griseofulvin 11 mg/kg/day PO div q24h × 4–8 wk
Black-dot ringworm	
Gray-patch ringworm	
Tinea corporis	Topical clotrimazole, miconazole or tolnaftate bid × 4 wk
Tinea cruris	Topical (as above) × 4–6 wk
Tinea pedis	Topical (as above) × 6–12 wk; oral griseofulvin for *Trichophyton rubrum*
Onychomycosis	Oral griseofulvin × 3–4 mo
Candidiasis	
Thrush	Nystatin PO 200,000 U qid × 6–12 days
Diaper rash	Oral nystatin *PLUS* nystatin cream qid

FEVER

Much more important than fever per se is its underlying cause. Once this has been determined, antipyretics may be used for the child's comfort and to help prevent febrile convulsions in the susceptible age group. Newer pharmacokinetic data offer better guidelines for administration of acetaminophen or aspirin.

TABLE 4-13. ANTIPYRETIC THERAPY

Acetaminophen	Loading dose: 22 mg/kg
	Maintenance: 13 mg/kg q6h
Aspirin	Loading dose: 18 mg/kg
	Maintenance: 8.5 mg/kg q6h

FEVER OF UNKNOWN ORIGIN (FUO)

A working diagnosis of FUO is convenient for classification of children who have had a temperature above 38.4C for more than 21 days and who have been adequately evaluated for the more common causes of fever. Prognosis for children with these criteria is much better than for adults who are much more likely to have a malignancy or autoimmune process as the cause of prolonged fever.

Children with FUO warrant an extensive evaluation directed primarily at less common causes of fever. Only one-third of cases however, are resolved by delineation of unusual etiologies as outlined in Table 4-14. One third represent confusing presentations of common disorders, which later become apparent, whereas one third will remain undiagnosed although these patients subsequently become afebrile and asymptomatic.

TABLE 4-14. ETIOLOGIES OF FUO

Unusual presentations of common diseases
  UTI
  Upper respiratory infection
  Infectious mononucleosis
  Sinusitis
  CMV
  Toxoplasmosis
  Pneumonia
  Meningitis
  Allergic disorders
  Dehydration
  Rheumatic fever
Infectious diseases
  Tuberculosis
  Osteomyelitis
  Septic arthritis
  Salmonellosis
  Hepatitis
  Tularemia
  Endocarditis
  Abdominal abscess
  Liver abscess
  Brucellosis
  Leptospirosis
  Malaria
  Relapsing fever

Autoimmune
  JRA
  SLE

Malignancies
  Leukemia
  Lymphoma
  Neuroblastoma
Miscellaneous
  Crohn's disease
  Factitious
  Drug fever
  Sarcoidosis

The most rewarding aspect of diagnostic evaluation is a meticulous history and physical examination. Laboratory studies should be guided by these or by prior screening data to avoid unnecessary, invasive, or expensive procedures. A suggested workup is presented in two phases (Table 4-15). The first phase includes a broad screen of diagnostic possibilities, which should be obtained on all patients. The second phase includes invasive procedures, which should only be undertaken if the clinical situation appears more urgent. It is best to proceed in a sequential fashion during these latter investigations.

TABLE 4-15. EVALUATION OF FUO

Phase one
  CBC
  Sedimentation rate
  Urinalysis and culture × 2
  TB skin test
  EB virus titer
  Chest x-ray
  Blood culture
  ASO titer
  Lumbar puncture (young infant)
  ANA
  Salmonella O and H antibodies
Phase two
  Hospitalize for observation
  Repeat blood cultures
  Sinus and mastoid x-rays
  Ophthalmologic examination for iridocyclitis
  Serologic tests for
    CMV
    Toxoplasma
    Hepatitis A and B
    Tularemia
    Brucella
    Leptospirosis
  Liver enzymes
  Abdominal ultrasound
  Upper GI with follow through

TABLE 4–15. (continued)

Bone marrow
Technetium bone scan
Abdominal CT scan

OROPHARYNGEAL INFECTION

Almost all "upper respiratory infections" are caused by viral agents and require only symptomatic therapy. Pharyngitis or tonsillitis without nasal involvement is more commonly associated with group A streptococci and a throat culture or test for streptococcal antigen is essential for determining this bacterial etiology. Often, documentation of an outbreak of oropharyngeal infection caused by a particular viral pathogen offers guidance to management of subsequent cases. Rare but important bacterial pathogens causing pharyngitis are *Neisseria gonorrhoeae*, *Corynebacterium diphtheriae*, and *Francisella tularensis* with other groups of streptococci, particularly C and G, accounting for isolated outbreaks of disease.

**TABLE 4-16. UPPER RESPIRATORY
INFECTIONS—COMMON ETIOLOGIC AGENTS
AND TREATMENT**

Classification	Etiology	Treatment
Common cold	Rhinovirus Parainfluenza RSV	Symptomatic
Nasopharyngitis	Adenovirus Enteroviruses (e.g., herpangina) Rhinoviruses Parainfluenza Influenza RSV	Symptomatic

(continued)

TABLE 4-16. (continued)

Classification	Etiology	Treatment
Pharyngitis–tonsillitis	Viruses (as with naso-pharyngitis)	
	Bacteria	
	Group A streptococci	Penicillin
	Streptococci (groups C and G)	Penicillin
	N. gonorrhoeae	Penicillin
	F. tularensis	Streptomycin
Peritonsillar abscesses	Group A streptococci	Penicillin
	S. aureus	Nafcillin
		Incision and drainage

OTITIS EXTERNA (SWIMMER'S EAR)

Otitis externa is caused by retention of water in the external canal with resulting bacterial replication and inflammation. Recovered bacterial pathogens are those which commonly colonize skin and thrive in moist environments.

TABLE 4-17. ORGANISMS CAUSING OTITIS EXTERNA

S. aureus
Pseudomonas aeruginosa
Proteus vulgaris
Streptococcus pyogenes
Enterobacteriaceae

Therapy is directed at eradication of probable organisms with broad spectrum topical antibiotics which can be accomplished with a brief (5 to 7 day) course. Children who swim frequently or have had repeated bouts of otitis externa should instill an acidified alcohol solution into the external canals after swimming or showering.

TABLE 4-18. TREATMENT OF OTITIS EXTERNA

Acute treatment (tid × 5–7 days) otic drops
   Cortisporin (polymyxin B, neomycin, and hydrocortisone)
   Otobiotic (polymyxin B and hydrocortisone)
Prophylaxis (swimmer's ear drops) after swimming or showering

OTITIS MEDIA

Otitis media is the most common outpatient diagnosis with a bacterial etiology made in pediatric practice. The incidence is between 10% and 20% for each year of life up to age 6 and then decreases dramatically to less than 1% by age 12. By definition these patients require antimicrobial therapy and therefore this diagnosis accounts for the greatest volume of antibiotic prescription writing. It is imperative for the physician to acquire the necessary skills and employ strict criteria for this diagnosis.

Viruses are rarely primary pathogens in middle ear infections and the various bacteria recovered by tympanocentesis are limited to organisms that commonly colonize the nasopharynx. Disease is the consequence of the eustachian tube in infants being relatively wider and shorter than in older children thereby allowing ready colonization of the middle ear with potential pathogens.

TABLE 4-19. ETIOLOGY OF OTITIS MEDIA IN INFANTS AND CHILDREN

S. pneumoniae	50%
H. influenzae	25%
Group A streptococci	15%
Branhamella catarrhalis	7%
S. aureus	2%
Others	1%

The antibiotic of choice for otitis media remains amoxicillin at a dose of 20 to 40 mg/kg/day (maximum 750 mg) divided q8h for 10 days. Patients who are apparent therapeutic failures or who relapse should undergo diagnostic tympanocentesis rather than an empiric change in antibiotic therapy. Most will yield sterile middle ear fluid thereby demonstrating adequacy of antimicrobial treatment.

Bacteria causing otitis media in the first 6 weeks of life include gram-negative coliforms, which are frequently resistant to amoxicillin. A diagnostic tympanocentesis is therefore required to guide therapy. In addition, these patients should be carefully evaluated for evidence of systemic disease including meningitis.

TABLE 4-20. ETIOLOGY OF OTITIS MEDIA IN NEONATES

Gram-negative enterics	
(*E. coli, Klebsiella, Pseudomonas, Proteus*)	60%
H. influenzae	15%
S. pneumoniae	15%
S. aureus	15%
Others	10%

PARASITIC INFECTIONS

Most parasitic diseases have virtually disappeared in developed countries as a result of concentrated efforts to improve sanitary conditions. Only pinworm (enterobiasis) and giardiasis are seen with any frequency in pediatric practice with occasional cases of ascariasis, amebiasis, strongyloidiasis, toxocariasis, hookworm, and whipworm (trichuriasis) requiring management. This section includes only these more common parasites. Giardiasis and amebiasis are discussed in Chapter 8 because they present with predominantly gastrointestinal symptoms.

TABLE 4-21. PRESENTING MANIFESTATIONS OF COMMON PARASITIC INFECTIONS

Pinworm	Perianal pruritis
Ascariasis	Passage of adult worms
Strongyloidiasis	Marked eosinophilia
	Immunosuppression
	Diarrhea
Toxocariasis	Marked eosinophilia
	Visceral larval migrans
Hookworm	Usually asymptomatic anemia
Whipworm (trichuriasis)	Chronic diarrhea

The most common parasitic disease, pinworm, probably should not be treated, primarily because reinfection is almost universal. The presence of *Enterobius* is also of minor clinical consequence. Most important is reassurance of the family that these nematodes are not the result of poor hygiene.

Strongyloides infection in the immunocompromised patient is associated with a high degree of parasitemia, dissemination, and significant mortality even with early administration of thiabendazole.

TABLE 4-22. TREATMENT OF MORE COMMON PARASITIC INFECTIONS

Pinworm	Pyrantel pamoate 11 mg/kg (maximum 1 g)
	Mebendazole 100 mg bid × 3 days (treat all household members)
Ascariasis	Pyrantel pamoate 11 mg/kg (maximum 1 g)
	Mebendazole 100 mg bid × 3 days
Strongyloidiasis	Thiabendazole 50 mg/kg/24 hr div q12h × 2 days

(continued)

TABLE 4-22. (continued)

Toxocariasis	Thiabendazole 50 mg/kg/24 hr div q12h × 1–4 wk (depending on symptoms)
Hookworm	Mebendazole 100 mg bid × 3 days
Whipworm (trichuriasis)	Mebendazole 100 mg bid × 3 days

Unusual parasitic infections are more likely to be seen in immigrants and individuals who have traveled to endemic areas. Presenting symptoms are commonly diarrhea, weight loss, rash, eosinophilia, skin ulcers, or fever. Many of the drugs of choice are only available from the Parasitic Disease Drug Service, Centers for Disease Control (CDC), Atlanta, Ga. Telephone consultation may be obtained by calling (404) 452–4174.

TABLE 4-23. TREATMENT OF UNUSUAL PARASITIC INFECTIONS

	Drugs Available Commercially
Malaria (except *Plasmodium falciparum*)	Chloroquine 20–25 mg of base/kg total dose (maximum 1.5 g) in 4 doses div 0, 6, 24, and 48 hr with the first dose being twice that of subsequent doses *PLUS* Primaquine phosphate 0.3 mg of base/kg (maximum 15 mg) qd × 14 days (first test for G6PD deficiency)
P. falciparum	Quinine sulfate 20 mg of the salt/kg (maximum 650 mg) div tid × 14 days *PLUS* Pyrimethamine 0.6 mg/kg (maximum 50 mg) qd × 3 days *PLUS* Sulfadiazine 50 mg/kg (maximum 2 g) div qid × 5 days
Schistosomiasis	Praziquantel 60 mg/kg single dose

TABLE 4-23. (continued)

Tapeworms	
Diphyllobothrium latum	Niclosamide 30 mg/kg
Taenia saginata and *T. solium*	Niclosamide (maximum 2 g) single dose
Hymenolepis nana	Niclosamide 30 mg/kg (maximum 2 g) qd × 5 days
Trichinosis	Thiabendazole 50 mg/kg/day div bid × 7 days
	Drugs available from CDC
Chagas' disease	Nifurtimox
Dracunculiasis	Niridazole
Leishmaniasis	Pentostam
Onchocerciasis	Suramin
Trypanosomiasis	
T. brucei gambiense	Pentamidinine
T. brucei rhodesiense	Suramin
CNS infection	Melarsoprol

RABIES PROPHYLAXIS

Postexposure rabies management has become much easier now that immunotherapeutic agents of extremely low toxicity have become available. Rabies immune globulin is prepared from the plasma of human volunteers hyperimmunized with rabies vaccine thereby eliminating serum sickness episodes so common with animal rabies serum, and human diploid cell vaccine is not associated with the encephalitic reactions so characteristic of duck embryo vaccine. The only drawback to this present treatment is the high cost.

TABLE 4-24. POSTEXPOSURE RABIES MANAGEMENT

Routine treatment of animal bites (see Table 4-7)
Rabies management
    Healthy domestic animal: observe animal for 10 days
    Wild rodent (mouse, rat, rabbit, squirrel, etc.): rarely is rabies
      prophylaxis indicated

(continued)

TABLE 4-24. (continued)

Wild animal (skunk, raccoon, bat, fox, etc.) or escaped domestic
  animal (dog or cat):
    HRIG 20 IU/kg total dose
      10 IU/kg infiltrated around wound
      10 IU/kg IM
    HDCV
      1 ml IM on days 0, 3, 7, 14, and 28
      Follow-up rabies antibody titer on day 42

SNAKEBITES

Most snakebites are inflicted by nonpoisonous species or result in
minimal envenomation where pit vipers (rattlesnakes, water
moccasins, and copperheads) are involved. Simple observation
for progression of local or systemic symptoms during a 4-hour period following the bite is the only therapy usually required. Coral
snake bites should always be considered potentially fatal. Large
rattlesnakes and water moccasins account for the largest number
of serious or fatal bites. The greatest number of poisonous bites,
however, are inflicted by copperheads, which are small and whose
bites almost never result in fatal consequences. A conservative
approach is therefore indicated when this species is identified.

TABLE 4-25. EMERGENCY TREATMENT
OF SNAKEBITES

Apply tourniquet loosely, proximal to edema
Splint
Transport to medical facility
For large snakes where transport will take > 1 hr
  Clean the bite
  Make 5 mm incision over fang marks
  Apply suction
  DO NOT
    Use tight tourniquet
    Pack on ice

Initial assessment of the patient is directed at determining the amount of envenomation and time lapse between the bite and institution of definitive therapy. Antivenin therapy should be started within 2 hours of the bite to assure maximum benefit. Guidelines for amount of antivenin are detailed in the package insert. Surgical consultation should be obtained if the bite is on a distal extremity because a fasciotomy may become necessary to preserve neurovascular function.

TABLE 4-26. IN-HOSPITAL TREATMENT OF SNAKEBITES

Admit for observation
Laboratory studies
  CBC, U/A, electrolytes
  Blood type and crossmatch
  Clotting studies monitored frequently
Antivenin IV for significant envenomation
  Begin within 2 hr of bite
  Skin test for hypersensitivity
  Dose is individualized
    Moderate cases—3-5 vials
    Severe cases—10-20 vials
    Children—relatively higher doses
  Monitor for allergic reactions
  Serum sickness common at 4-7 days
Fasciotomy if neuromuscular function compromised
Tetanus prophylaxis
Severe cases
  Volume expanders, respiratory support, dialysis

5

Procedures

ASPIRATE OF CELLULITIS

Needle aspiration of the leading edge of an area of cellulitis should be obtained for culture, particularly when *Haemophilus influenzae* is a suspected pathogen. The area should be cleansed with an iodine solution and washed with alcohol. A 22- or 23-gauge needle is attached to a syringe containing 0.5 ml of normal saline *without* bacteriostatic preservative. The needle is advanced 1 cm into superficial subcutaneous tissue, the saline injected and aspirated back into the syringe. The syringe and its contents should be transported to the laboratory for direct plating on appropriate media. Blood culture bottles should not be used because these do not contain adequate growth nutrients for *H. influenzae* and other organisms.

BLADDER TAP

The procedure is carried out with the patient lying supine and the lower extremities held in the frog leg position. The suprapubic area is cleansed with iodine and alcohol, and the symphysis pubis is located with the index finger. Using a 20-ml syringe and a 22-gauge, 1½-inch needle or 2-inch spinal needle in older children, the abdominal wall and bladder is pierced in the midline about 1½ to 2 cm above the symphysis pubis. The needle is then angled 30 degrees toward the fundus of the bladder. Urine is gently aspirated and the needle withdrawn. No dressing is necessary. As with the venipuncture, neither sterile gloves nor local anesthesia is required in doing vesicopuncture.

BLADDER WASHOUT

At present, a bladder washout is the best procedure for localizing UTIs. Performed properly, data correlate almost absolutely with those from ureteral catheterization, a much more invasive procedure. Patients must be restrained during bladder washout, nursing personnel should be well trained, and collected urine samples must be carefully labeled as to time and sequence of collection.

TABLE 5-1. BLADDER WASHOUT METHODOLOGY

Restrain patient
Catheterize bladder with a Foley catheter
Empty bladder and submit for urinalysis and culture #1
Instill 75 ml of 2% neomycin in normal saline plus 2 amps of Elase; clamp catheter for 45 min
Empty bladder; irrigate bladder with 2 L of distilled water in 50 ml aliquots; submit last irrigation for culture #2
Collect urine q10min × 5 and submit each for culture (#3–#7)

TABLE 5-2. BLADDER WASHOUT INTERPRETATION

Cystitis
  Negative cultures after irrigation
Pyelonephritis
  Progressive increments in colony counts
      #1 is positive
      #2 is negative
      #3–#7 (>100 colonies/ml), 10-fold increase from #3 to #7

BLOOD CULTURE

For those infectious processes where bacteremia is associated, blood cultures represent an important source for etiologic diagnosis. These specimens are essential particularly during the initial workup of sepsis, meningitis, endocarditis, pneumonia, cellulitis, osteomyelitis, and septic arthritis. Only one culture is necessary in neonates and young infants because the density of bacteria is higher and the bacteremia more continuous than in older patients. After age 12 months, two cultures should be obtained and for endocarditis, three to six are recommended.

TABLE 5-3. BLOOD CULTURE TECHNIQUE

Wash hands
Clean rubber stopper of culture bottle with alcohol
Clean skin with 2% iodine or Betadine
Wipe skin with alcohol
Perform venipuncture without touching puncture site
Obtain 1–5 ml of blood
Change needles aseptically
Transfer blood to bottles (aerobic and anaerobic)
Volume of sample: a 1:10 to 1:20 dilution (2.5 to 5 ml for 50-ml
  culture bottle) for routine cultures; 1:50 (1 ml) is adequate for
  Bactec methodology

CENTRAL LINE QUANTITATIVE CULTURES

Often it is difficult to determine whether a catheter is the source of septicemia, particularly if there are other potentially infected sites. Although removal of an indwelling catheter is usually simple and provides a definitive diagnosis in catheter-related sepsis, it may be undesirable to remove permanent catheters from patients who have a limited number of sites for infusion or whose parenteral hyperalimentation central lines are the only source of nutrition. Quantitative blood cultures performed with the catheter in place can be compared to quantitative cultures of peripheral blood, thereby establishing whether the catheter is the source of infection and therefore must be removed.

TABLE 5-4. PROCEDURE FOR QUANTITATIVE BLOOD CULTURES

Notify laboratory to provide 2 empty sterile petri dishes and 2 melted TSA deeps (in a beaker of hot water)
Flush catheter with 10–20 ml of saline
Aseptically draw 2–6 ml of blood from the catheter and from a peripheral vein
Using a tuberculin syringe, place 0.1 ml of blood from each site in a separate petri dish
Pour TSA over the blood and swirl the dish to evenly suspend the blood
Allow agar to harden and transport to laboratory
Process the remaining blood as for routine blood cultures
Interpretation: quantitative counts from the catheter that are >10-fold those of peripheral blood indicate catheter infection

LUMBAR PUNCTURE

CSF should be examined in any child where meningitis is suspected. The only absolute contraindications to lumbar puncture are increased intracranial pressure or a mass lesion of the CNS. In such cases a CT scan should first be obtained. Other relative contraindications are anticoagulation, platelet count of less than 20,000, meningomyelocele, severe scoliosis, or suspected abscess in the lumbar area. Always perform a fundoscopic examination, obtaining a clear view of the optic disc prior to performing a lumbar puncture.

TABLE 5-5. TECHNIQUE FOR LUMBAR PUNCTURE

Restrain patient in recumbent or upright position (upright preferred
  for neonates who may have very low CSF pressure)
Scrub hands, wear surgical gloves and mask
Locate L3–4 interspace at the level of the iliac crest
Clean the back thoroughly with an iodine solution, wash with
  alcohol or wipe dry
Drape with sterile towels
Insert a 22-gauge spinal needle (B bevel) in the L3-4 interspace,
  directed toward the umbilicus
Remove the stylet periodically or when the "pop" of the dura is felt
If blood returns, the procedure may be repeated in the L2–3
  interspace.

LUNG ASPIRATION

Needle aspiration of the lung is the most useful direct method for
establishing the etiology of pneumonia in children. Because this
procedure is associated with a 1 to 5% incidence of pneumo-
thorax, it should not be undertaken unless determining the causative pathogen would alter therapeutic approaches. Such
circumstances are most commonly a severely ill or immune compromised host, suspicion of an unusual organism, or failure of response to initial empiric therapy.

TABLE 5-6. NEEDLE ASPIRATION OF THE LUNG

Determine with x-ray the major site of involvement
Clean skin with an iodine solution, wash with alcohol
Use sterile gloves; sterile towels are rarely necessary
Anesthetize skin and soft tissue down to pleura (2% procaine) above
  a rib
Attach a 22-gauge spinal needle (B bevel) to a 10-ml syringe
  containing 1 ml of normal saline without bacteriostatic
  preservative
Time puncture to maximum inspiration; if possible have patient
  pause in inspiration for 3–4 sec

(continued)

TABLE 5-6. (continued)

Rapidly advance needle into lung 3 cm, directed toward the hilum,
  maintaining negative pressure with the syringe; the aspiration
  should take only 2 sec
Transport needle, syringe, and their contents to the laboratory for
  inoculation into enrichment broth or direct plating

OSTEOMYELITIS SUBPERIOSTEAL ASPIRATION

Needle aspiration of suspected osteomyelitis should be a routine
initial procedure for etiologic diagnosis. This will not alter interpretation of subsequent bone scans and there is no risk of intro-
ducing disease into bone if there is an overlying area of cellulitis.

TABLE 5-7. TECHNIQUE FOR SUBPERIOSTEAL ASPIRATION

Clean skin with an iodine solution; wash with alcohol
Drape area with sterile towels; use sterile gloves
Anesthetize skin only
Using a syringe containing 0.5 ml of normal saline, aspirate
  subcutaneous tissue as for cellulitis
Using a second 2.5-ml syringe and 20-gauge needle, advance the
  needle until the bone is touched and aspirate (saline is not needed)
Transport the needle and syringe to the laboratory for direct plating

PERICARDIOCENTESIS

Though pericardiocentesis may be done in most any setting as an
emergency, under ideal conditions it is best done in an intensive
care unit or cardiac catheterization laboratory (where fluoroscopic control is possible). Constant ECG monitoring is essential and
constant or frequent BP monitoring is also important.

   The patient is placed in a supine position with the head and
chest elevated slightly. The area of the xiphoid is properly

prepped and draped. Using sterile technique, the skin and subcutaneous tissue at and just to the left of the xiphoid are infiltrated with a local anesthetic. With a syringe attached, an 18- or 20-gauge needle of 5 to 10 cm length is inserted adjacent to the xiphoid (in the notch between the xiphoid process and the seventh costal cartilage) and advanced slowly toward the middle of the left clavical. The needle is kept at an angle of 20 degrees off the skin. The needle is passed immediately posterior to the costal cartilage and as it passes through the pericardium a "pop" may sometimes be felt.

An exploring electrode (V lead) may be attached to the metal hub of the needle with a sterile alligator clamp and the ECG so monitored. A "current of injury" pattern is noted as the pericardial space is entered and the epicardium encountered.

Constant negative pressure is kept on the syringe as the needle is advanced, and pericardial fluid is aspirated as soon as the needle perforates the pericardium. As much fluid as possible should be removed, but in the presence of suppurative pericarditis, the purulent material may be difficult to aspirate or may be loculated.

If bloody fluid is obtained, set aside a small sample in a glass tube to observe. Blood that has been in the pericardial space for any significant time will not clot. Blood aspirated from the cardiac chamber will clot normally. Check the hemoglobin content and hematocrit of the fluid aspirated to compare with the patient's peripheral blood values. If the heart has been perforated, remove the needle slowly and observe the patient's vital signs frequently. Perforation of the inferior surface of the right ventricle has rarely resulted in persistent bleeding into the pericardial space.

Some physicians prefer to use a needle–plastic cannula set so that once the pericardial space is entered, and the needle is slipped out of the plastic cannula covering it, and fluid is then aspirated via the cannula. This technique may be safer if a large quantity of fluid is to be removed and considerable time is required to remove it. These plastic cannulas, however, may be stiff enough to perforate the heart of a small child, so great care must still be exercised in manipulating the cannula in the pericardial space.

PERITONEAL TAP

An abdominal paracentesis should be accomplished when primary peritonitis is suspected. Most cases of peritonitis secondary to a perforated viscus require surgery when appropriate cultures are obtained.

TABLE 5-8. PROCEDURE FOR PERITONEAL TAP

Empty urinary bladder
Sedate patient
Place patient in supine position
Clean skin over rectus muscle with iodine from symphysis pubis to
  umbilicus
Anesthetize skin, soft tissue, and peritoneum just lateral to midline
  in the lower third between symphysis pubis and umbilicus
Make 5 mm incision in skin
Assure aseptic technique
Using #14F abdominal trocar, insert through incision directed
  obliquely up and back; continue advancing until release through
  the peritoneum is felt
Remove stylet and collect fluid for culture, gram stain, and cell
  count
Suture incision and apply sterile pressure dressing

SUBDURAL TAPS

Subdural effusions occurring during or after therapy for bacterial meningitis can be detected clinically by enlarging head circumference, split sutures or fontanels, and lateralizing findings on neurologic examination. Effusions can be evaluated by skull roentgenograms, transillumination of the skull and CT scan. Subdural fluid aspiration, when indicated, is easily done on infants with open fontanels. Adequate immobilization of the child is necessary. After shaving the scalp widely around the anterior fontanel, sterile prepping and draping of the scalp, and surgical gloving, an 18- to 20-gauge subdural needle with stylet is introduced into the lateral recess of the anterior fontanel at the coronal suture. Anesthetic agents are generally not required in infants. The subdural needle is introduced 3 to 5 mm through the dura and the stylet removed. Subdural fluid may well from the needle. If no subdural fluid is encountered, suctioning and probing of the subdural space generally is not recommended. Occasionally by rotating or withdrawing the needle and reintroducing it at a slight angle under the convexity of the skull, flow may be established. A thick exudate of purulent empyema or markedly elevated subdural fluid protein may account for lack of flow. Similarly, loculated fluid beyond the reach of the subdural needle may be present. In these cases, a CT scan may be necessary to exclude the possibility of loculated subdural empyema or ventricular enlargement clinically suggesting subdural effusions. If subdural fluid flow is established, 20 to 30 ml of fluid may be removed, and routine studies including cell count, glucose, protein determination, and gram stain are done. Bilateral subdural taps are indicated in some cases. In general, subdural taps, if done without probing, are innocuous; however, occasionally trauma to the cerebral cortex, bleeding into the subdural space, and prolonged leakage of subdural or subarachnoid fluid following subdural tap may occur. Proper antiseptic preparation precludes infection. Indications for repeated subdural taps are controversial and these increase the risk of fistula formation and iatrogenic infection. The ready availability of CT scans has decreased the indications for subdural fluid aspirations and permitted a more accurate evaluation of effusion size and localization.

THORACENTESIS

Thoracentesis is performed both for diagnosis and therapeutic purposes. For empyema caused by *H. influenzae*, pneumococcus, or group A streptococci, one or two thoracenteses will often provide adequate drainage, thus avoiding placement of a chest tube.

Empyema, as a result of *Staphylococcus aureus*, almost always necessitates chest tube drainage.

TABLE 5–9. PROCEDURE FOR THORACENTESIS

Place patient in sitting position
Clean skin with iodine solution; wash with alcohol
Anesthetize skin, soft tissue, and pleura in 7th or 8th interspace (level of the tip of the scapula), posterior axillary line
Drape with sterile towels; use surgical gloves
Use 18-gauge needle attached to a 3-way stopcock and syringe; enter pleural cavity above a rib
Remove fluid for culture, gram stain, and chemistries (see Table 6–16)
Obtain postthoracentesis chest x-ray
If patient begins coughing, remove needle immediately
If no fluid is obtained, consider repeating under fluoroscopic direction

TYMPANOCENTESIS

This procedure should be considered for any neonate with otitis media where gram-negative coliform bacteria are commonly recovered, and for older patients who have persistent signs and symptoms of middle ear disease after standard therapy.

TABLE 5–10. ASPIRATION OF MIDDLE EAR FLUID

Remove cerumen
Clean canal with alcohol
Culture external ear canal to monitor contaminants
Restrain patient
Use an 18-gauge, 3½-inch spinal needle bent at a double angle (as a fork) attached to a 2.5-ml syringe
Use an otoscope with an operating head
Advance needle through a speculum that has been sterilized in alcohol
Penetrate the posterior–inferior aspect of the tympanic membrane
Aspirate middle ear exudate and transport to laboratory for culture and gram stain

VENTRICULAR TAP

Ventricular taps are generally performed by neurosurgeons; however, the procedure may be useful or mandatory in some emergency situations or in cases where CSF must be obtained without lumbar puncture prior to beginning antibiotic therapy. Sterile surgical technique is used in all cases. In infants, the ventricular system can be entered by inserting a spinal or ventricular needle through the lateral aspect of the anterior fontanel at the coronal suture, directing the needle toward the midpoint of the orbit on that side. In older children, a burr hole can be drilled in the mid-pupillary line at the hairline and the needle introduced. Obviously, these facial landmarks vary and experience and a clear mental image of the ventricular system are needed prior to attempting a ventricular tap. The return of clear or blood-tinged CSF documents correct needle aspiration. Pressure measurements are obtained and sufficient fluid drained both for diagnostic purposes and at times, therapeutic effect. CT and cranial ultrasound are useful in accurately judging the need for and the effects of ventricular tap and should be routinely performed.

VENTRICULOPERITONEAL SHUNT ASPIRATION

Because of the wide variety of shunts currently used in neurosurgery, the surgeon responsible for following the patient's shunt should generally be contacted before aspiration is attempted. Some shunt systems have sites designed for safe aspiration. In other cases, skull radiographs reveal shunt characteristics that help identify the model and specific mechanics. In cases where shunt patency or possible infection is questioned, shunt aspiration is an uncomplicated and safe procedure if sterile technique is used. The goal of the procedure should be not only to obtain CSF, but also to document proximal and distal patency. After shaving the bulb site, a surgical scrub is performed and sterile drapes and gloves used. A 23-gauge butterfly needle and catheter is preferred. CSF flow suggests proximal patency. By elevating the catheter and using a manometer, if necessary, ventricular pressure can be measured. Elevating the catheter and noting drainage of CSF suggests distal patency. Rarely is the quantity of fluid obtained critical. Sufficient fluid should be obtained liberally to carefully and thoroughly perform all cytologic, chemical, and microbiologic cultures and smears (including large amounts of fluid if fungal studies are indicated). Following removal of the needle, CSF may leak and the site should have a sterile dressing and be observed for infection. In general, if the bulb site itself appears infected, no aspiration should be attempted.

BODY SURFACE AREA

For some patients, antibiotic dosages should be based on body surface area (see Table 18–15). Using the general reference information on the following page (Figure 5–1), determine the point of intersection on the surface area for a line drawn through the patient's height and weight.

General Reference Information

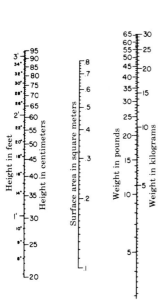

Surface area sq cm = $wt^{0.25} \times ht^{0.725} \times 1.84$

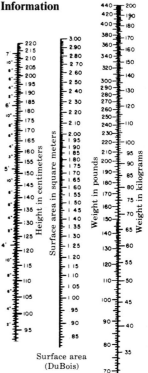

Surface area
(DuBois)

SURFACE AREA AND WEIGHT

Approximate relation, in individuals of average bodily proportions:

Weight		Area	Weight		Area
kg	lb	M²	kg	lb	M²
2	4.4	0.12	25	55	0.93
3	6.6	0.20	30	66	1.07
4	8.8	0.23	35	77	1.20
5	11	0.25	40	88	1.32
6	13	0.29	45	99	1.43
7	15	0.33	50	110	1.53
8	18	0.36	55	121	1.62
9	20	0.40	60	132	1.70
10	22	0.44	65	143	1.78
15	33	0.62	70	154	1.84
20	44	0.79			

6

Laboratory Diagnosis

The clinical laboratory is continually striving to meet the needs of both the attending physician and the patient by providing prompt and accurate results. Accomplishing this goal in the most proficient manner necessitates good communication and cooperation between the physician and the laboratory technologist. This chapter attempts to provide the clinician with a simplified review of the available laboratory tests to provide information from which to base clinical decisions.

It is the responsibility of the physician to ensure that an appropriate and properly collected specimen is obtained from the patient and promptly delivered to the laboratory. Upon receipt, the submitted specimen will be inspected to determine if it is of sufficient quality and quantity for adequate evaluation.

STAINS

Microscopic examination of unstained and stained smears of specimens from an infected site is the most direct, rapid, and least technical of procedures.

Gram Stain

Gram-positive and gram-negative organisms are differentiated on the basis of the cell wall and cell membrane permeability characteristics to organic solvents. These characteristics are probably due to the glycosaminopeptide and lipoprotein composition of the bacterial cell wall. Gram-positive organisms, which do not have significant amounts of lipid as an integral part of their cell wall, retain the crystal violet-iodine complex and stain purple, whereas gram-negative organisms do not retain this complex and stain red from the counterstain.

TABLE 6-1. GRAM STAIN

Specimen source: Most clinical specimens
Technique
  Air dry smear and fix with methanol (allow to evaporate)
  Flood slide with crystal-violet (60 sec)
  Wash, add Gram's iodine (60 sec)
  Decolorize with acetone alcohol (5 sec) and wash immediately
  Counterstain with safranin (15 sec)

TABLE 6-1. (continued)

Staining identification
  Gram-positive organisms stain purple
  Gram-negative organisms stain red

Acid-fast Stain

This stain should be performed if pulmonary tuberculosis or tuberculous meningitis is suspected. It is based on the observation that the staining of mycobacteria with carbol fuchsin resists decolorization with acid alcohol. Other acid-fast organisms such as *Nocardia* sp. may also be detected using this procedure, but must be identified further with special stains and cultures. A technique using auramine and rhodamine fluorescent dyes is easier to read although it is more time consuming compared to the acid-fast stain.

TABLE 6-2. ACID-FAST STAIN

Specimen source
  Sputum
  CSF
Technique
  Air dry and fix with methanol (allow to evaporate)
  Flood slide with Kinyoun carbol-fuchsin (4 min)
  Wash with water and decolorize with acid
    alcohol until faint pink
  Wash, counterstain with methylene blue (30 sec)
Identifying organisms
  Acid-fast (stain red)
    Mycobacteria sp.
    Nocardia sp.
  Nonacid-fast bacteria and cellular elements stain blue

Methylene Blue Stain

Methylene blue is a useful stain to establish the morphology of organisms and to differentiate cells found in the specimen (neutrophils, lymphocytes, monocytes, RBCs, and epithelial cells). Intracellular bacteria, such as *Neisseriae*, are often more evident with this stain as are other bacterial characteristics as demonstrated by the capsules surrounding pneumococci and the metachromatic granules of *Corynebacterium diphtheriae*.

Wright's and Giemsa Stains

Both Wright's and Giemsa stains are extremely helpful in demonstrating organisms, inclusion bodies, or cellular differentiation in various specimens.

TABLE 6–3. USES OF WRIGHT'S AND GIEMSA STAINS

Used to stain
    Intracellular organisms in blood (buffy coat)
    Conjunctival scrapings
    Impression smears
    Tissue sections
Used to differentiate
    Multinucleated giant cells in vesicle fluid of herpes virus skin or
        mucosal infections (see Tzanck Preparation)
    Cell types (PMNs, lymphocytes and trachomatis inclusions,
        eosinophils, epithelial cells, monocytes)
Used to detect
    Rickettsiae
    Chlamydiae
    Protozoa (malaria)
    Selected yeast and fungi

WET MOUNTS

Unfixed samples can be examined microscopically as wet mounts for bacterial, fungal, parasitic, and other pathogens (Table 6-4). These commonly used wet mounts are: normal saline, used to detect trichomonads and protozoa; potassium hydroxide (KOH), used primarily for identification of fungal forms; and india ink mounts for identifying encapsulated *Cryptococcus*.

TABLE 6-4. THREE COMMONLY USED WET MOUNTS

Normal Saline	KOH	India Ink
Specimen source		
Cervical secretions	Cervical discharge	CSF
Vaginal secretions	Skin scrapings	Urine
Urethral discharge	Sputum	Exudates
Urine sediment	Tissue scrapings	Sputum
Feces		
Technique		
Mix 1–2 drops of 0.9% NaCl and examine microscopically	Mix 1 drop 10% KOH, allow to stand 10–15 min and examine microscopically	Mix 1 drop of India ink and examine microscopically
Identifying organisms		
Trichomonas vaginalis	Fungal forms	Capsule of *Cryptoccocus neoformans* (must see budding yeast)
Protozoa (trophozoites, cysts of *Entamoeba histolytica*)		
Pinworm eggs		

SPECIMEN EXAMINATION AND ANALYSIS

Cerebrospinal Fluid (CSF)

Collection of CSF is performed under sterile conditions and divided into three 1-ml aliquots for microbiologic cultures, chemistry determinations, and cell counts. A fourth sample may be obtained for viral cultures.

TABLE 6-5. PROCESSING CSF FROM MENINGITIS PATIENTS

Sample Aliquot	Diagnostic Tests	Volume
1	Culture Bacteria (and fungi)	1.0–2.0 ml
2	Protein and glucose (compare with simultaneous blood glucose)	1.0 ml 1.0 ml

(continued)

TABLE 6–5. (continued)

Sample Aliquot	Diagnostic Tests	Volume

3	Total WBC and RBC count
	Sediment for staining
	   Wright's stain cell differential
	   Gram stain (80% positive in meningitis)
	   Acridine orange for rapid detection of
	    bacteria
	   Acid-fast stain
	   India ink (other fungal stains)
	Antigen detection (CIE, CoA, etc.)
		1.0 ml

In the bacteriologic examination of CSF the gram-stained smear is an extremely important rapid identification of meningitis. It normally takes approximately 1 to 10×10^4 bacteria per milliliter before detection by a direct smear is possible. Centrifugation of the CSF at 2000 rpm for 10 minutes increases the precentage of positive smears made from the sediment. Caution must be taken because of artifacts staining similarly to organisms.

TABLE 6–6. COMMON ERRORS IN CSF STAINING INTERPRETATION

Gram stain
   Confusing precipitated stain as gram-positive cocci
   Identifying false capsules because of poor stain
   Misreading of *H. influenzae* with bipolar staining as
    overdecolorized pneumococci
India ink preparation
   Cells or artifacts that appear to be *Cryptococcus* sp. causing
    false-positive results

Dark-field examination for spirochetes, if syphilitic or leptospiral meningitis is suspected, is available in most laboratories as well as a variety of rapid immunologic assays that are capable of demonstrating the type-specific polysaccharide capsule antigens of pneumococcus, meningococcus, and *H. influenzae* (see Table 6-21).

Urine

The laboratory aid to the diagnosis of a UTI is only as valid as the care given to the collection of a urine specimen for culture and examination. Consequently, the method of collection (see Chap. 10) of urine is important, and it is necessary to know how collection was accomplished in order to interpret results. The volume of urine recommended for a urinalysis is 15 ml or more but as little as 2 ml will suffice for a screen.

Microscopic examination of formed elements must clearly be identified to determine early diagnosis of urinary tract infection. This can be done with wet mounts and staining of urine sediment. Practically all uncentrifuged urine with bacterial colony counts of greater than or equal to 10^5/ml will have a positive gram stain. Several rapid screening methods are available for the identification of bacteriuria. Glucose and nitrite determinations by the dipstick technique to detect bacterial metabolism must be interpreted with caution because dilute urine will result in false-negative results. None of these tests have yet replaced bacterial cultures in the detection of UTIs.

TABLE 6-7. ROUTINE SCREENING URINALYSIS

Test	Volume
Screening for bacteriuria Gram stain of uncentrifuged specimen Quantitative loop culture	2–3 drops
Specific gravity (performed using a refractometer)	1 drop
Microscopic examination of sediment RBCs, leukocytes, renal epithelial cells, hyaline casts, mucous and excess crystals, microorganisms	1 drop of concentrated sediment

(continued)

TABLE 6-7. (continued)

Test	Volume

Basic chemical screen (tested with a multiple or single reagent strip)
  pH (≥ 7.5 in infection)
  Blood
  Protein
  Bilirubin
  Glucose
  Urobilinogen
  Ketone
  Nitrite
	2 ml

An important aspect of evaluating a patient with suspected UTI is to identify the organism with routine and quantitative cultures.

TABLE 6-8. BACTERIOLOGIC CULTURES FOR URINE

Routine cultures
  Blood agar
  MacConkey agar or EMB for gram-negative bacilli
  TSA
Special considerations
  Pyuria in the absence of bacterial growth by routine culture
  might indicate the possible presence of *Mycobacterium*
  tuberculosis. Sediment from the first morning specimen should
  be Gram stained and cultured

Quantitative urine cultures may be obtained by using bacteriologic loops that deliver approximately 0.001 and 0.01 ml of a sample of urine. A sterile loop is dipped into urine from a properly collected specimen and streaked on a blood agar plate. After incubating 18 to 24 hours at 37C the number of colonies of bacteria on the blood agar plate is multiplied by 1000, giving a reasonable approximation of the bacteria per milliliter in the urine specimen. Thus more than 100 colonies on a plate is evidence of significant bacteriuria and a quantitative colony count of 10^5 colonies per milliliter.[3]

Urine obtained directly by bladder puncture or catheterization is normally sterile and any growth of urinary pathogens should be considered significant.

Fecal Specimens

Fecal specimens should be collected and transported in paper stool cups. Care should be taken not to contaminate the stool with urine or water because of the possibility of killing trophozoites. The guaiac method represents a suitable test for routine screening of blood in stool.

TABLE 6-9. EVALUATION OF FECAL SPECIMENS

Gross examination
  Consistency, odor, presence of blood, pus, undigested food, mucus, parasites
Microscopic examination
  Fecal leukocytes stained with methylene blue or Wright's stain
  Ova and parasites (wet mounts and Scotch tape prep)
Routine cultures—Fecal specimens are routinely cultured for *Staphylococcus aureus*, *Salmonella*, *Shigella*, *Campylobacter*, and *Yersinia*. It is worth noting that enteropathic *E. coli*, *Vibrio* sp. and viruses require special handling and media
  Blood agar
  MacConkey or other selective media for gram-negative enteric bacilli
  HE agar, Selenite, SS agar for *Salmonella* and *Shigella*
  GN (gram-negative) broth
  CVA plates for *Campylobacter*

TABLE 6-10. GUAIAC METHOD FOR OCCULT BLOOD

Place about 0.5 g of feces into a test tube
Add 2 ml of water and mix
Add 0.5 ml glacial acetic acid and guaiac solution
Mix 2 ml 3% H_2O_2 with suspension
Observe for 2 min and note maximal blue intensity as 1^+, 2^+, 3^+, or 4^+
Green denotes a negative test

TABLE 6-11. STAINING PROCEDURE FOR FECAL LEUKOCYTES

Place small fleck of mucous or stool on glass slide
Add 2 drops of Loeffler's methylene blue and mix
Wait 3 min and examine under low power
Make a rough quantitative count by approximating average number of leukocytes and erythrocytes
Differential is performed under high power

A predominance of PMNs is seen with any inflammatory enterocolitis.

TABLE 6-12. FECAL LEUKOCYTES ASSOCIATED WITH GI DISEASES

Disease	Average Predominant Leukocyte
Salmonellosis (other than *S. typhi*)	75% PMNs, 25% mononuclear cells
Typhoid fever	95% mononuclear cells
Shigellosis	84% PMNs
E. coli (invasive)	85% PMNs
Ulcerative colitis (active)	88% PMNs, 8% eosinophils
Amebic dysentery (active)	Commonly mononuclear cells, unless secondary bacterial infection
Viral diarrhea, cholera, and healthy controls	—

Ova and Parasites

When parasitism is highly suspected, a minimum of three specimens should be submitted. The major parasitic species that infect the intestinal tract are protozoa and helminths. The protozoa (amebiasis and giardiasis) have two major forms, trophozoite and cyst. Inspection of the perianal area at night, after the child is asleep, may reveal adult pinworms (thread-like white worms ¼ to ½ inches).

TABLE 6-13. SIMPLE METHODS FOR DETECTING PARASITES

Direct wet mounts
    Place fleck of stool on glass slide
    Add 2 drops of 0.9% NaCl for trophozoites and ova or 2 drops of iodine stain for cysts
Scotch tape preparation for pinworm
    Obtain preparation immediately after child awakens
    Cover one end of a tongue depressor with cellophane tape (sticky side out)
    Apply to perianal area with mild pressure
    On a glass slide place one drop of xylol and then transfer tape to slide
    Examine for ova under microscope

Synovial Fluid (SF)

SF aspiration may provide information to distinguish between the joint inflammation due to infectious, immunologic, or traumatic involvement. The specimen should be collected using sterile technique to avoid contamination from exogenous birefringent material. Ideally, the patient should be fasting for 6 to 12 hours to allow equilibrium of glucose between plasma and SF. Infected SF tends to clot spontaneously or within an hour, therefore specimens to be examined microscopically for cells and bacteria should be placed immediately into a heparinized tube.

TABLE 6-14. EVALUATION OF SYNOVIAL FLUID

Gross examination	Color, turbidity, viscosity, clotting (observe clot formation after 1 hr), organisms, crystals
Cell counts	Enumerate WBC and RBC
Stains	Wright's stain, gram stain (65% positive in bacterial infected SF), methylene blue, acid-fast stain
Glucose	SF glucose level is usually <50% of the blood glucose level in septic arthritis. Levels may be normal particularly in gonococcal arthritis
Mucin	Normal SF forms tight cordlike coagulum clump in 5% acetic acid that is stable for 24 hr. Fluid from infected joints results in poor unstable mucin clot
Cultures	Routine cultures include blood agar, nutrient broth supportive of anaerobes, and chocolate agar or Thayer-Martin for gonococcus. Special consideration for *M. tuberculosis*, fungi, or viral agents
Immunologic tests	CIE is helpful in detecting antigens of *H. influenzae* and *S. pneumoniae*, especially during antibiotic treatment

TABLE 6-15. EXAMINATION OF SYNOVIAL FLUID

Test	Normal and Noninflammatory	Severe Inflammatory	Infectious–Septic
Color	Clear straw	Yellow to opalescent	Yellow to green
Clarity	Transparent	Opaque [a]	Opaque
Viscosity	High	Low	Variable
WBC/mm^3	0–5000	500–50,000	500–200,000
Neutrophils	<25%	>50%	≥75%
Culture	Negative	Negative	Positive [b]
Mucin clot	Firm	Slightly friable to friable	Friable

TABLE 6-15. (continued)

Test	Normal and Noninflammatory	Severe Inflammatory	Infectious–Septic
Glucose (blood-SF difference in mg/dl)	0–10	0–40	20–100

[a] Monosodium urate crystals in gout or calcium pyrophosphate dihydrate crystals in pseudogout may be found.

[b] Postive in about 50% because of low virulent organisms or partially treated.

Pleural, Pericardial, and Peritoneal Fluids

It is important to differentiate these fluids as to whether they are transudates, caused by mechanical factors influencing formation, or exudates that may be caused by infection due to damage of the mesothelial linings.

TABLE 6-16. DIFFERENTIATING TRANSUDATES AND EXUDATES

Pleural fluids (PF)
    90% exudates >3 g/dl total protein
    80% transudates <3 g/dl total protein
    >95% of pleural exudates have at least one of the following
      characteristics (>95% PF transudates have none of the findings)
      Protein/serum protein (ratio >0.5)
      LDH/serum LDH (ratio >0.6)
      LDH >600U
      Specific gravity > 1.016
      pH < 7.2
Peritoneal fluid
    Total protein 2–2.5 g/dl to separate transudates from exudates

TABLE 6-17. EVALUATION OF FLUID EXUDATES

Gross appearance (color, clarity, odor)
Total WBC and RBC counts
Differential (Wright's stain) or cytologic study
Gram stain
Culture (blood agar, medium selective for gram-negative bacilli,
  EMB anaerobic and aerobic growth, and chocolate agar for *H. influenzae*)
Chemistry (total protein, LDH, glucose)

CULTURES
Care must be emphasized for proper specimen collection to avoid or minimize unnecessary contamination.

Blood Cultures
Whenever there is a reason to suspect clinically significant bacteremia, a blood culture should be ordered. The necessity for strict aseptic technique in the course of obtaining blood for cultures should be stressed. A newer method using the BACTEC 460 system has recently been introduced to the clinical laboratory. The BACTEC 460 is an instrument used to test inoculated BACTEC blood culture vials for the presence of liberated radioactive carbon dioxide ($^{14}CO_2$). Should a high level of $^{14}CO_2$ be present in a vial, it indicates that there are living microorganisms that originated in the initial inoculum. All cultures are read on the BACTEC each day for 7 days. All positive bottles, whether they be aerobic or anaerobic, are subcultured aerobically unless the gram stain shows a possible anaerobe.

The aerobic subculture should include a blood chocolate biplate, and if gram-negative rods are seen on gram stain, a MacConkey plate should be set up also. The anaerobic subculture, if done, should include a reducible blood plate and a CNA-LKV biplate.

Anaerobic Cultures
Many anaerobic bacteria of clinical importance are fastidious and oxygen intolerant. Special anaerobic containers must be used in

specimen collection and transport. Rapid processing of samples also is important in avoiding overgrowth by facultative anaerobes.

Fungal Cultures

Scrapings, hairs, or other specimens are planted on Sabouraud agar and incubated for 2 to 4 weeks at room temperature. Positive cultures are examined microscopically by one of the three common wet mounts described in Table 6–4.

Viral Cultures

Several innovative methods for the rapid identification of viral infections have been developed because of the renewed interest in useful viral diagnoses. The etiology of a viral syndrome may often be established by viral culture, serologic tests, or both. Table 6–19 outlines the type of specimen necessary for the isolation of a virus from various clinical syndromes. The serologic methods recommended for viral agents are noted in Table 6–21.

TABLE 6-18. GENERAL PROCEDURES FOR VIRAL SPECIMEN COLLECTION

1. Specimens should be obtained early in the course of illness, when virus shedding is greatest, preferably within 3 days, and generally no later than 7 days after the onset of symptoms.
2. The type of specimen and clinical syndrome should be clearly recorded, because different processing steps prior to attempted isolation are necessary for different types of samples, and only certain viruses are found in some specimen types.
3. Samples collected on swabs (conjunctival, pharyngeal, nasopharyngeal, rectal) should be placed quickly in a liquid virus transport medium provided by the laboratory.
4. Because many viruses are heat labile, samples should be placed in sterile containers, packed in wet, crushed ice, and transported promptly to the virology laboratory. Many specimens can be held at 4C for up to 24 hr (on wet ice or in a refrigerator) without significant decrease in recovery. For prolonged storage, specimens should be frozen at −70C.

(continued)

TABLE 6-18. (continued)

Specimen guidelines
1. Nasal secretions. A calcium alginate swab is introduced through the anterior nares into the nasopharynx and plunged into the transport medium after removal from the nares. Nasal washings are collected by instilling 4–5 ml of infusion broth into each nostril while the patient extends the neck slightly and closes the posterior pharynx (by pushing against "k" sound). The head is tilted forward and a sample collected in a clean container held beneath the nose.
2. Pharynx. A swab of the posterior pharynx should be taken by touching the swab to both tonsillar areas and to the posterior pharyngeal wall.
3. Blood. Citrated whole blood, 3–5 ml, can be used to isolate viruses from the buffy coat (e.g., HSV, rubella).
4. CSF. Collect 1–3 ml into a sterile container and process immediately. Avoid freezing particularly for cytomegalovirus.
5. Urine. Collect 5–10 ml of a clean catch, midstream urine into a sterile container and process immediately.
6. Feces. Place a 2–5 sample into a clean specimen container without transport medium. A rectal swab is less satisfactory but can be obtained by inserting a cotton-tipped swab stick 5 cm into the rectum and gently rotating the swab. In contrast to rectal cultures for gonococcus, some fecal material should be obtained when doing viral studies.
7. Vesicular fluid. After decontamination of overlying skin, aspirate the lesion with a Pasteur pipette, or a small-gauge needle attached to a tuberculin syringe, or open the vesicle and collect fluids and cellular elements from the base onto a swab. If a crust is present, the crust should be lifted off; the fluid beneath the crust then can be swabbed (see Tzanck Preparation below).

Tzanck Preparation. The Tzanck preparation is done to distinguish between pustular pyodermas and vesicular lesions due to herpes virus. Scrapings obtained from the base of a vesicle are air dried onto a glass slide and stained with Wright's stain. Smears demonstrating multinucleated giant cells with central aggregation of nuclei and/or intracytoplasmic inclusions strongly suggest herpes infection.

**TABLE 6-19. COLLECTIONS FROM SUSPECTED
VIRAL INFECTIONS**

Syndrome	Source of Specimen for Viral Isolation	Most Common Agents
Upper respiratory tract infection	Nasal wash or nasopharynx	Rhinovirus Parainfluenza 1,3 RSV Adenovirus 1, 2, 3, 5, 14, 21
Lower respiratory tract infection		
Child	Nasal wash	RSV
	Nose or throat swab	Parainfluenza 3, 1, 2
	Sputum	Influenza A
Adult		Influenza A
Pleurodynia	Throat swab	Coxsackie A, B
	Stool	
CNS infection		
Meningitis	CSF	Mumps
	Throat swab	Coxsackie A, B
	Stool	ECHO
Encephalitis	Blood	Mumps Herpes simplex I
Myocarditis and pericarditis	Throat swab Stool	Coxsackie B
Gastroenteritis	Stool	Norwalk, Hawaii agents Reovirus
UTI		
Acute hemorrhagic cystitis	Urine	Adenovirus 2, 7, 11 and ECHO 9
Orchitis and epididymitis	Throat swab Stool	Mumps
Parotitis	Throat swab Stool	Mumps
Exanthemata (nonspecific, with fever)	Skin vesicle fluid Throat swab Stool	Coxsackie A9, A16 ECHO 9, 16, 11
Herpangina	Skin vesicle fluid Throat swab Stool	Coxsackie A (1–6,8,10,16,22) Coxsackie B

(continued)

TABLE 6-19. (continued)

Syndrome	Source of Specimen for Viral Isolation	Most Common Agents
Hand-foot-and mouth disease	Skin vesicle fluid Throat swab Stool	Coxsackie A
Nonspecific febrile illness	Nose and throat swab Stool Blood	Coxsackie A, B ECHO Influenza A, B

Chlamydia Culture

Presumptive evidence of *Chlamydia* can be obtained by the examination of stained smears (Giemsa) for the presence of inclusions. Most laboratories today employ cell culture procedures for the isolation of *Chlamydia*. After inoculation and incubation, the cells are stained with iodine (see Stains in this chapter). Antibodies to *C. trachomatis* are usually accomplished by CF (group specific) or micro-IF (immunotype-specific) methodology.

Table 6–20. SPECIMENS AND TESTS USED FOR CHLAMYDIA IDENTIFICATION

Chlamydia	Specimen	Tests
C. trachomatis	Urethral swabs Cervical scrapings Posterior nasopharyngeal Tracheal secretions Conjunctival scrapings	Giemsa stain, cell cultures, serology ELISA, CIE, IHA (IgM is diagnostic in infants)
C. psittaci	Respiratory secretions Conjunctival scrapings Biopsy of lung (postmortem)	

ANTIMICROBIAL SENSITIVITY TESTING

Antimicrobial sensitivity testing should be performed only when pathogens have unpredictable susceptibility patterns to the commonly used antibiotics. Sensitivities are not routinely performed on group A streptococci or *Neisseria* sp. because they have relatively predictable susceptibility patterns to antibiotics.

The methods available for sensitivity testing include disc diffusion (agar diffusion), agar dilution (plate dilution), and broth dilution (tube or microtiter plate dilution).

Disc Diffusion Testing

The Kirby-Bauer disc diffusion method is the most commonly used antimicrobial susceptibility test. The technique requires the inoculation of an agar plate with a standard inoculum, addition of disk containing a standardized quantity of antimicrobial agent, incubation for 18 hours, and measurement of the zones of inhibition. A three-category system of reporting results of disc diffusion testing is often used: sensitive, intermediate, and resistant.

Dilution Susceptibility Testing

Dilution susceptibility tests are used to determine the minimal inhibitory concentration (MIC) and minimum bactericidal concentration (MBC) of an antibiotic for an infecting organism. The MIC of the drug is defined as the lowest concentration that prevents visible growth of the test organism under a standardized set of conditions. The MBC of the drug is the lowest concentration that results in complete killing (99.9%) of the test organism. The MIC and MBC are expressed quantitatively in micrograms, international units, or micromoles of antibiotic per milliliter. Dilution susceptibility testing can be done by a broth dilution or agar dilution method.

β-Lactamase Test

The development of rapid assays for β-lactamase permits an assessment of sensitivity to penicillin or ampicillin before standard disc diffusion of broth dilution susceptibility testing results are available. Rapid acidometric, iodometric, and chromogenic cephalosporin methods currently are used to detect β-lactamase production. Bacteria can be tested after overnight growth in media, and results are usually available within 30 minutes to an hour.

Successful therapy of infections caused by *Haemophilus influenzae, Staphylococcus aureus,* and *N. gonorrhoeae* may be facilitated by knowing whether the infecting agent is sensitive or resistant to penicillin or ampicillin. Resistance is correlated with the production of the enzyme, β-lactamase.

SEROLOGIC AND IMMUNOLOGIC TESTING

Serologic methods are employed to detect microbial antigen as rapid diagnostic tests or to determine host antibody responses to suspected pathogens. Because of the nature of the immune response patients generally are 10 to 12 days into their clinical illness before most serologic tests are able to measure a response. For conclusive evidence of infection, usually either a conversion from negative to positive or a fourfold rise in titer must be demonstrated. In some cases the titer will decrease. An acute phase serum and a convalescent serum (2 to 4 weeks after the onset of the infection) should be submitted to the laboratory.

TABLE 6–21. COMMONLY USED SEROLOGIC TESTING FOR INFECTION

Disease	Source of Specimen	Serology Test	Comment
Bacterial infections			
Syphilis	Blood	VDRL, RPR, ART	Titer should decrease with successful treatment
		FTA-ABS	Titer remains elevated after successful therapy
	CSF	VDRL	Positive titer in CSF uncontaminated with blood is indicative of neurosyphilis. *Note:* FTA-ABS should not be ordered on CSF specimen
Group A streptococci	Blood	Streptozyme, ASO	Titer ≥ 1:300 is suggestive of recent infection
Pneumococcal, meningococcal or *H. influenzae* type B meningitis	CSF	CIE CoA or latex agglutination	
Group B streptococci	CSF Blood/ CSF	Latex agglutination	
Legionnaire's disease	Blood	CIE Indirect fluorescent antibody	Fourfold rise in IF titer to ≥ 1:128 indicative of recent infection. Single titer ≥ 1:256 may also indicate recent infection

(continued)

TABLE 6-21. (continued)

Disease	Source of Specimen	Serology Test	Comment
Mycoplasma pneumoniae		CF Cold agglutinins	Fourfold increase in titer Nonspecific IgM antibody response; may not appear until after acute phase of infection
Salmonella Brucellosis Rickettsial infections Tularemia	Blood	"Febrile agglutinins"	
Fungal infections Cryptococcal meningitis	CSF	Latex agglutination	
Histoplasmosis Coccidioidomycosis	Blood Blood	CF CF, precipitins	
Parasitic infections Amebiasis	Blood	IHA (indirect hemagglutination)	Test most sensitive for extraintestinal infection; less sensitive for intestinal infection
Toxoplasmosis	Blood	IFA (indirect fluorescent antibody)	Fourfold rise in antibody titer

Chlamydia			
Trichinosis	Blood	ELISA IHA, FA Bentonite flocculation	Test does not usually detect antibody before 3rd or 4th wk after ingestion of parasite. A titer of 1:5 or more of a fourfold rise suggests infection
Viral infections			
Hepatitis B	Blood	RIA (radioimmunoassay) for hepatitis surface antigen and antibody to core antigen	
Hepatitis A	Blood	ELISA RIA	IgM antibody rise is consistent with recent infection. IgG antibody represents prior infection
Influenza	Blood	CF	Fourfold rise
Adenovirus	Blood	CF, ELISA	Fourfold rise
Mumps	Blood	CF	Fourfold rise
Rubella	Blood	HI, ELISA	Fourfold rise, acute IgM levels can be tested
Measles	Blood	CF, HI, neutralization, ELISA	Fourfold rise
CMV	Blood	CF, ELISA Cytologic IgM	Fourfold rise
HSV	Blood	Neutralization, CF, ELISA	
EBV	Blood	ELISA	Fourfold rise, may not be seen in recurrent infection

149

7

Respiratory Infections

Respiratory tract infections constitute a major problem for the pediatrician, accounting for an estimated 30 to 40% of all office visits. The manifestations of the majority of infections are limited to the upper respiratory tract (i.e., ears, nose, throat), but as many as 5% may involve the lower respiratory tract. It should be emphasized that although the symptoms of a respiratory tract infection are fairly well localized, pathologic and physiologic changes may be widespread. A frequent example of this is the acute exacerbation of asthma (lower airway involvement) triggered by a common cold.

Greater than 90% of respiratory infections are viral in origin (excluding otitis media). Difficulty in documenting etiology of an infection has led to indiscriminate antibiotic use. Fortunately, the age of the patient, the localization of the symptoms, and the status of the host's defenses help predict the organism and the need for antimicrobial therapy. For a large proportion of bacterial infections, an underlying alteration in host defenses can be postulated.

TABLE 7-1. AGE-RELATED ETIOLOGY OF LOWER RESPIRATORY TRACT INFECTIONS

	Virus	Bacteria	Mycoplasma	Other
Premature and newborn	+	+++	−	
Early infancy	+	+	−	+++[a]
Infancy	++++	+		
Toddlers	+++	+++	−[b]	
5–10 years	+++	+	++	
>12 years	+	+	++++	

[a] Afebrile pneumonia group.
[b] Frequent cause of common cold.

PNEUMONIA

The majority of acute pneumonias are viral with probably less than 10% bacterial. Pneumonia can be difficult to distinguish from atelectasis radiographically, but is usually diagnosed on the basis of cough, fever, dyspnea, tachypnea, and crackles in association with an infiltrate on the chest film. Histologically, pneumonia is inflammation and exudate of the alveoli and alveolar walls. Pneumonia has been characterized as interstitial or alveolar based on its radiographic appearance, but this description is only vaguely helpful in formulating a differential diagnosis. Bacterial pneumonia (i.e., pneumococcus, *H. influenzae*, and *Staphylococcus*) frequently have a segmental distribution whereas viral infections tend to be diffuse and interstitial. Neutropenic patients may suffer from pneumonitis with very little evidence of infiltrate on chest x-ray. The only reliable way to differentiate viral from bacterial pneumonia is positive identification of an organism(s), which may require a lung biopsy. Other supporting evidence for bacterial pneumonia is rapid onset, highly toxic appearance, fever of more than 39C, leukocytosis with a high proportion of neutrophils, and parapneumonic effusion or empyema. Supporting evidence for a viral pneumonia includes concomitant systemic complaints (i.e., myalgia, diarrhea, photophobia), only mild temperature elevation, little toxicity, and a relatively increased proportion of lymphocytes in the peripheral blood.

Tables 7–2 and 7–3 list the more common etiologic organisms. Ideally, therapy should be tailored to the specific organism, and every reasonable effort should be made to make the correct identification (see Table 7–4). For the critically ill patient who is progressing to respiratory failure despite therapy, it is necessary to proceed promptly to an emergency open lung biopsy. This can be performed safely even in the most critically ill patient. Open lung biopsy often affords a rapid diagnosis based on histology and specific stains. Newer methods of rapid diagnosis should be utilized when available (see Chap. 6).

Respiratory syncytial virus (RSV) is the major cause of bronchiolitis and is a frequent cause of pneumonia in infancy; rhinovirus is a more frequent cause of pneumonia in school-aged children. Influenza A and B, parainfluenza, and adenovirus tend to occur in epidemic fashion.

TABLE 7-2. VIRUSES CAUSING LOWER RESPIRATORY TRACT INFECTION

Organism	Pneumonia	Bronchiolitis
RSV	++	++++
Influenza (A and B)	++	+
Parainfluenza	++	++
Adenovirus	+++	+
Rhinovirus	++	++

++++ = most frequent; + = occasional.

TABLE 7-3. CHARACTERISTICS OF BACTERIAL PNEUMONITIS

	Pneumo-coccus	H. influenzae	Staphylococcus
Age	Infancy	Infancy	Infancy
High fever	++++	++++	++++
WBC >15,000	++++	++++	++++
Chest x-ray	Segmental or lobar	Segmental or lobar	Segmental or lobar
Pleural effusion	+	++	++++
Positive blood culture	++++	++++	++

The etiology of segmental or lobar pneumonia in the toxic-appearing infant and young toddler is likely to be *Streptococcus pneumoniae*, *H. influenzae* (H. flu), or *Staphylococcus aureus* (Staph). It is not possible to distinguish between these on clinical grounds. In recent years *H. influenzae* has become a more frequent cause with relatively less frequent isolation of *Staphylococcus* observed. Children with *H. influenzae* pneumonia are at risk of other associated serious infections such as meningitis and purulent pericarditis. In all age groups outside of the neonatal period, *S. pneumoniae* is probably the most common cause of bacterial pneumonia.

TABLE 7-4. STANDARD DIAGNOSTIC METHODS FOR PNEUMONIA

Test	Bacteria	Virus	Other
Throat swab		+	
Rectal swab		+	
Serology	+	+	+
Urine culture		+	
Blood culture	+		

TABLE 7-4. (continued)

Test	Bacteria	Virus	Other
Sputum culture	+		
Sputum stains	+		+
Sputum cell count	+		+
Thoracentesis	+		
Bronchoscopy	+		+
Lung puncture	+		+
Open lung biopsy	+	+	+

Mycoplasma

Mycoplasma pneumoniae is an organism that has features of both bacteria and viruses. Community serologic surveys indicate that mycoplasma is a frequent cause of the common cold in the preschool-age group. In older school-age children and adolescents, it is probably the most common cause of pneumonia. Radiographically there may be a segmental or lobar infiltrate(s) and the patient seems less ill than the chest x-ray would indicate. On occasion mycoplasma pneumonia is life-threatening and may involve many other organ systems; patients with sickle cell anemia may be particularly prone to severe infection. The diagnosis should be made by culture or specific serology. Cold agglutinins are specific but not a sensitive laboratory test; ready availability, however, makes this a useful screening procedure.

Granulomatous

Pneumonia with organisms that form granulomas (i.e., *Mycobacterium tuberculosis*, *Histoplasma capsulatum*, *Coccidioides immitis*, *Blastomyces dermatitidis*) generally occur in endemic areas, whereas other organisms in this group generally occur in immunocompromised patients (*Candida albicans*, *Aspergillus fumigatus*, *Cryptococcus neoformans*). The diagnosis can generally be made by culture when the appropriate organisms are suspected and

sought. If skin testing is to be done, serum for fungal titers should
first be obtained. In certain endemic areas, it may be difficult to
separate acute infection from previous infection based on skin
testing and serology; this would include the Mississippi and Ohio
river valleys for histoplasmosis and the southwestern United
States for coccidioidomycosis. In healthy persons, infection with
this group of organisms is usually mild and unrecognized. In
compromised patients, it is often fatal (see Chap. 16).

**TABLE 7–5. ORGANISMS CAUSING
GRANULOMATOUS PNEUMONIA**

M. tuberculosis
H. capsulatum
C. immitis
B. dermatiditis
C. albicans
A. fumigatus
C. neoformans

Afebrile Pneumonia of Infancy

A new class of pneumonitis is being recognized more frequently
in afebrile neonates and infants. Etiologic organisms are listed in
Table 7-6. Mixed infections are common. Infection is acquired by
delivery through a colonized birth canal. The clinical presentation is tachypnea, poor weight gain, and inspiratory crackles;
fever and wheezing are uncommon. The chest x-ray usually
shows hyperaeration, peribronchial thickening, and scattered
areas of atelectasis. The diagnosis should be made by culture or
histologic examination of sputum or lung. Chlamydia is suggested by eosinophilia, elevated immunoglobulins, and clinically
by the presence of conjunctivitis. A specific IgM antibody titer
can confirm this etiology. Treatment includes erythromycin 50
mg/kg/day divided q6h for 14 to 21 days.

TABLE 7-6. ORGANISMS CAUSING AFEBRILE PNEUMONITIS OF EARLY INFANCY

Chlamydia trachomatis
Cytomegalovirus
Pneumocystis carinii
Ureaplasma urealyticum

Necrotizing Pneumonia

Necrotizing bacterial pneumonia is not a common pediatric problem. Patients at risk are usually debilitated, immunocompromised, and have been hospitalized for a long time. Patients treated with broad spectrum antibiotics may develop pneumonia with an organism that is resistant to multiple antibiotics. Organisms causing necrotizing pneumonitis are *Pseudomonas aeruginosa*, *Klebsiella pneumoniae*, *Proteus mirabilis*, and related species. Each hospital tends to have its own predominant organism with a specific sensitivity pattern. Despite aggressive antibiotic therapy, pneumonias with this group of organisms is often fatal.

TABLE 7-7. ORGANISMS CAUSING NECROTIZING PNEUMONITIS

P. aeruginosa
K. pneumoniae
P. mirabilis
Enterobacter sp.
Serratia marcescens
Escherichia coli
Acinetobacter calcoaceticus

Aspiration Pneumonia

Pneumonia due to aspiration of gastric contents or oropharyngeal secretions occurs almost exclusively in patients with impaired neurologic function. A depressed level of consciousness, albeit transient, as in seizure disorders, induction of anesthesia, or diabetic coma, or permanent as in mental retardation, is a constant predisposing factor. Chronic aspiration also occurs frequently in patients with an uncoordinated swallowing mechanism. Careful history and physical examination should uncover the potential for aspiration pneumonitis. The organisms are usually anaerobes, and frequently more than one organism is isolated. The infiltrates on chest x-ray are usually in the dependent lobes; effusions and abscesses are common. The prognosis for complete recovery from the acute pneumonia is good with appropriate antibiotic therapy. Depending on the nature of the neurologic impairment, prevention of recurrent aspiration pneumonitis and permanent lung damage may be difficult.

TABLE 7-8. ORGANISMS CAUSING ASPIRATION PNEUMONIA

Peptostreptococcus
Peptococcus
Microaerophilic cocci and streptococci
Bacteroides sp.
Fusobacterium sp.
S. aureus
Streptococcus pyogenes
Streptococcus sp.

Legionnaires' Disease

The significance of the "new" pneumonias in pediatrics is not completely delineated. Legionnaires' disease, caused by *Legionella pneumophilia* and other *Legionella* species, is believed to be an uncommon cause of pneumonia in noncompromised children, but serologic studies suggest a large percentage of the population may have been infected during childhood and adolescence. Extrapolating from extensively studied epidemics in adults, pneumonia due to *Legionella* species is associated with high fever, prominent systemic symptoms (especially involving the gastrointestinal tract), and patchy densities on chest x-ray. The organism cannot be cultured on routine media; a presumptive diagnosis can be made by a titer of greater than 1:256 or a fourfold increase in titer. Immunofluorescent stains are available for making the diagnosis on biopsy specimens. Therapy with erythromycin generally brings prompt clinical improvement. The only other antibiotic seemingly effective is tetracycline, even though aminoglycosides and cefoxitin inhibit growth in vitro; this is probably due to the need for the antibiotic to penetrate the alveolar macrophage for therapeutic success in vivo.

Treatment
There is generally no treatment (except supportive) available or required for viral pneumonitis. Exceptions to this are amantadine or rimantadine for influenza, and acyclovir for Herpes simplex pneumonitis. Recent positive experience with inhaled ribavirin for RSV bronchiolitis may be extended to RSV pneumonitis in the future. Immunization is currently available for influenza and has been shown to prevent the illness or lessen its severity; all high-risk groups should be considered for immunization (see Table 3–5). It is common practice to prescribe oral antibiotics for patients who are mildly ill and have an infiltrate on the chest x-ray in the hope that any possible bacterial pneumonia will be adequately treated. Even with the high likelihood of viral pneumonia, the difficulty in delineating etiology coupled with the low toxicity of therapy, make it difficult to reprimand this practice.

TABLE 7–9. IV ANTIBIOTIC CHOICE FOR PRESUMED BACTERIAL PNEUMONIA

Age Group	Antibiotic[a]
<3 mo	Ampicillin *PLUS* methicillin IV *PLUS* cefotaxime, ceftriaxone, moxalactam or gentamicin (erythromycin if *Chlamydia* is suspected in infant <20 wk of age)

(continued)

TABLE 7-9. (continued)

Age Group	Antibiotic[a]
3 mo–5 yr	
Mild	Amoxicillin PO
Severe	Cefotaxime, ceftriaxone, or cefuroxime IV (add nafcillin if *S. aureus* is suspected)
5–10 yr	Penicillin PO or IV
10–21 yr	Erythromycin PO

[a] Dosage: see Tables 18-10, 18-11, 18-12, 18-13.

There is little question about the need for antibiotics in the toxic, febrile infant that appears to have bacterial pneumonia. All appropriate cultures, including thoracentesis fluid, should be obtained prior to starting them. Consideration should be given to hospitalization and intravenous administration of antibiotics effective against the suspected organism. Clinical improvement is generally rapid (within days) although radiographic improvement may take longer. Exudative effusions are commonly drained, but therapy of the underlying pneumonia is usually satisfactory therapy for the effusion as well. Some physicians recommend the use of closed tube thoracostomy drainage for parapneumonic effusions in an effort to prevent rind formation and restrictive lung disease. This seems to be an uncommon occurrence in the pediatric population and tube thoracostomy should be reserved for patients with a loculated or unresolving empyema (Chap. 14).

Antibiotics should also be considered for suspected mycoplasma pneumonitis, understanding that prompt resolution is not to be expected. Erythromycin and tetracycline are effective against mycoplasma. Infants with afebrile pneumonia are candidates for antibiotics after appropriate cultures have been obtained. Trimethoprim–sulfamethoxazole should be included in the regimen if *Pneumocystis carinii* is suspected and erythromycin or sulfisoxazole if chlamydia is suspected. Again, prompt resolution should not be anticipated.

IV antibiotics, usually an aminoglycoside in conjunction with a semisynthetic penicillin, are indicated for necrotizing pneumonia. Selection of particular antibiotics should be determined by organism sensitivities. The desired peak serum tobramycin or gentamicin level for appropriate treatment should be 8–12 μg/ml (a peak level represents the serum concentration 30 minutes after a 30-minute infusion); generally a 2.5 mg/kg dose or more given every 8 hours is required to achieve this peak. With normal renal function, a 6-hour dosing interval has been shown with pharmacokinetic data to be appropriate and safe in children. Survival and improvement are related to the underlying associated illness.

For aspiration pneumonia (as opposed to the chemical pneumonitis from hydrocarbon aspiration), penicillin or clindamycin is the drug of choice. Rarely a resistant *Bacteroides fragilis* will dictate the need for an aminoglycoside. Clinical improvement is usually prompt but radiographic improvement may be slower, especially if a parapneumonic effusion has been present.

TABLE 7-10. SHORT-COURSE CHEMOTHERAPY FOR NON-DISSEMINATED TUBERCULOSIS

1st mo	
Isoniazid	10–20 mg/kg (maximum 300 mg) qd
Rifampin	10–20 mg/kg (maximum 600 mg) qd
Subsequent 8 mo	
Isoniazid	20–40 mg/kg (maximum 900 mg) × 2/wk
Rifampin	10–20 mg/kg (maximum 600 mg) × 2/wk

Some supportive therapeutic modalities, although frequently used, have little scientific basis for their continued use. Supplemental oxygen should be considered to maintain the hemoglobin saturation greater than 90% (corresponding to a Pao_2 of about 60). If a decreasing pH suggests impending respiratory failure with respiratory acidosis or if adequate oxygenation cannot be maintained on safe amounts of oxygen, mechanical ventilation should be considered. Chest physical therapy and postural drainage do not speed recovery from pneumonia; it may be helpful if atelectasis is also present. Mist therapy has no benefit, although supplemental oxygen sources need some humidification. IPPB and inhaled mucolytics are of no benefit and may be contraindicated.

BRONCHIOLITIS

Bronchiolitis is a very common lower respiratory tract infection, affecting perhaps as many as 1 to 2% of all infants. About half of these infants require hospitalization. The peak ages range from 2 to 10 months. RSV is the predominant organism with other viruses being responsible in certain epidemics. The clinical manifestations are preceding coryza, cough, tachypnea, and wheezing. The chest x-ray shows hyperinflation, peribronchial thickening, and varying amounts of atelectasis. Histologically, there is mononuclear inflammation and sloughing of the bronchiolar epithelium with partial obstruction of the bronchiolar lumen.

TABLE 7-11. BRONCHIOLITIS

Age	2–10 mo
Organism	RSV predominates, adenovirus, parainfluenza
Symptoms	Wheezing and tachypnea
Therapy	Trial of bronchodilators: β_2 agonists (terbutaline 0.5 mg or metaproterenol 0.1 ml, each inhaled) or theophylline
	Supportive (O_2, etc.)
Sequelae	Recurrent wheezing
	Predilection for COPD

Therapy is primarily supportive with maintenance of adequate oxygenation and appropriate hydration and nutrition. A small percentage of infants will require mechanical ventilation. Antibiotics are not indicated as this is exclusively a viral illness. Chest physical therapy may be beneficial to those infants with atelectasis. Some infants seem to have less wheezing and a slower respiratory rate after administration of a bronchodilator such as subcutaneous epinephrine, inhaled terbutaline, or theophylline. Most retrospective studies have failed to show a more rapid recovery, however. A current trend is to administer a few doses of inhaled β_2 agonist looking for clinical improvement, and continuing therapy if there is a positive response. The antiviral agent ribavirin may be helpful in shortening the course of the illness and ameliorating the symptoms; additional studies are needed before this drug is available for widespread use. Steroids have not been beneficial in several large studies.

Although bronchiolitis seems to be a self-limited and a generally benign illness, the long-term sequelae may be significant. Up to 50% of the patients have subsequent wheezing or frank asthma. It is yet unclear what role small airway insults early in life have on chronic obstructive lung disease in adults. Some children appear to have asymptomatic small airways dysfunction years after the episode of bronchiolitis, suggesting a propensity for progressive dysfunction later in life.

BRONCHIECTASIS AND CYSTIC FIBROSIS

Bronchiectasis is the abnormal dilatation and destruction of the bronchial wall, and is the end result of different insults or systemic diseases. The etiology of bronchiectasis is changing as diseases such as pertussis and rubeola become less frequent and survival from systemic diseases improves. In some conditions, such as cystic fibrosis, the destruction is progressive, whereas in others, such as dyskinetic cilia, it is static. The symptoms suggesting bronchiectasis are productive cough, purulent sputum, foul smelling breath, and crackles or wheezes on examination.

TABLE 7-12. ETIOLOGY OF BRONCHIECTASIS

Cystic fibrosis
Pneumonia (e.g., adenovirus)
Dyskinetic cilia
Measles
Pertussis
Allergic bronchopulmonary aspergillosis
IgA deficiency
Hypogammaglobulinemia
Tuberculosis

Cystic fibrosis is the most common lethal genetic disease affecting Caucasian children, and death is usually due to progressive bronchiectasis and lung damage. The basic metabolic defect is unknown, but all exocrine glands are involved. The lung secretions are abnormally viscous, leading to plugging of the small airways. Subsequent inflammation and infection add to the volume and tenacity of secretions and produce the destructive enzymes that cause the tissue damage.

TABLE 7-13. CYSTIC FIBROSIS

Etiology	Unknown
Frequency	1/1500 live Caucasian births
	1/20 Caucasian are carriers
	1/10 as common in blacks
Genetics	Autosomal recessive
Affected systems	All; lungs and digestive predominate
Mean age of survival	21 yr (1982)

Colonization of the airways occurs early with *S. aureus*, changing to *P. aeruginosa* with increasing age. *Pseudomonas* is peculiar in that it tends to produce a mucoid coating. The organisms are seldom eradicated from the sputum with antibiotic therapy and if they are, they generally recur promptly. The colonization does not appear to be related to the patient's well-being or pulmonary status. The cystic fibrosis patient with these organisms in the sputum in no way resembles patients with staphylococcal or pseudomonas pneumonia. Nevertheless, traditional therapy for pulmonary exacerbations (i.e., increased dyspnea, sputum volume, sputum viscosity) has been tailored as though a staphylococcal or pseudomonas pneumonia is being treated. This generally consists of intravenous therapy with an aminoglycoside, a synergistic semisynthetic penicillin, and an antistaphylococcal penicillin for a period of 10 to 21 days.

TABLE 7-14. IV ANTIBIOTICS FOR CYSTIC FIBROSIS

Standard	Alternatives
Antistaphylococcal penicillin	
Oxacillin	First generation cephalosporin
Nafcillin	Erythromycin
Methicillin	Chloramphenicol
Aminoglycoside	
Gentamicin	Netilmicin
Tobramycin	Sisomicin
Amikacin	Third generation cephalosporin
Penicillin	
Carbenicillin	Azlocillin
Ticarcillin	
Piperacillin	

It has been documented that this approach improves the patient's well-being, chest x-ray appearance, pulmonary function, and gas exchange. Concomitantly there has been a progressive increase in the mean age of survival (now to 21 years). Nevertheless, which antibiotic regimen or what dosage is probably of little importance.

Also important in the acute therapy for cystic fibrosis patients is aggressive nutritional support and chest physical therapy.

Many cystic fibrosis patients have a reactive airways disease component and benefit from a bronchodilator. Mucolytics are used frequently but reports of any benefit are subjective only; N-acetylcysteine is irritating and may actually promote bronchospasm or additional inflammation.

Chronic home therapy of cystic fibrosis is also centered around antibiotics, nutrition, and chest physical therapy. It is not clear whether continuous antibiotic therapy is beneficial or if antibiotics should only be administered at times of increasing symptoms. Many children and young adults with moderate to severe disease seem to do better on continuous therapy. If chronic suppressant therapy is offered, an antistaphylococcal drug such as oxacillin or cephalexin is often chosen. The spectrum of coverage can be broadened by the addition of ampicillin, trimethoprim–sulfamethoxazole, cefaclor, erythromycin–sulfisoxazole, or tetracycline (older children only). None of these antibiotics is particularly active against *Pseudomonas* and occasionally oral carbenicillin is used; resistance often develops quickly, however. Probenecid may be used in an effort to increase serum penicillin levels.

Inhaled aminoglycosides (gentamicin or tobramycin) are increasingly popular for outpatient prophylaxis. Patients managed in this way seem to have fewer exacerbations and fewer hospitalizations. The combined use of inhaled and intravenous tobramycin has been used successfully in the hospital setting. Outpatient inhaled antibiotics will probably supplant the use of outpatient IM or IV therapy.

Transient bronchiectasis can occur after an episode of pneumonitis and occasionally bronchiectasis is permanent. This is fairly common after pertussis or rubeola, diseases that are becoming less frequent. Certain strains of adenovirus seem to cause severe disruption of the airways and may lead to bronchiectasis. Dyskinetic cilia and immunodeficiency syndromes lead to bronchiectasis with a pathogenesis similar to cystic fibrosis (i.e., recurrent infection and inflammation).

Medical treatment of noncystic fibrosis bronchiectasis consists of antibiotics and chest physical therapy. The antibiotic should be selected by sputum culture results if at all possible. As in the cystic fibrosis patient, it is not known whether antibiotics should be used continuously or intermittently. If the bronchiectasis is limited to a specific lobe or segment as documented by bronchography, and if the patient does not have a systemic disease that may cause bronchiectasis in other areas, surgical resection should be considered. Resection has been performed in the past in an effort to prevent the spread of bronchiectasis from one lobe to another, but this has probably reflected undiagnosed systemic disease rather than contiguous spread. Bronchodilators may be beneficial in some patients.

LARYNGOTRACHEOBRONCHITIS (LTB)

LTB is the most common cause of acute partial upper airway obstruction in children. The terminology describing this disease and those in its differential diagnosis (Table 7–15) has been confusing. LTB (or croup) refers to partial airway obstruction due to a viral infection with erythema and edema concentrated mostly in the subglottic area. The organism is usually parainfluenza (types 1, 2, 3), although other organisms can cause croup in an epidemic fashion (RSV, influenza, rhinovirus). The peak ages are between 6 months and 3 years. The clinical presentation is that of a child with a few days of upper respiratory tract infection who then develops inspiratory stridor, retractions, and a harsh barking cough. The degree of fever depends on the organism and is usually mild with parainfluenza. The severity of the obstruction is variable throughout the day and is often worse at night. The illness gradually resolves spontaneously over several days. No laboratory test is needed for confirmation but neck x-rays show characteristic subglottic narrowing. Therapy at home is symptomatic (i.e., antipyretics for fever) and mist. In-hospital therapy might include mist, oxygen, and racemic epinephrine (1:4 concentration of 2.25%, with increasing concentration to 1:1 as needed) by inhalation. Because of the potential for rebound, the use of racemic epinephrine commits the patient to further observation. The mixture of helium and oxygen is less dense than air and oxygen, and may be helpful in decreasing the need for vigorous respiratory efforts in children with upper airway obstruction.

It is uncommon for croup to require intubation. Because edema and inflammation are in the narrowest portion of the child's airway, a somewhat narrower endotracheal tube should be selected to decrease the likelihood of postintubation subglottic stenosis.

Spasmodic croup occurs in the slightly older child and is probably a variant of reactive airway disease rather than an infection, although a viral disease may predispose the child to spasmodic croup. Characteristically the previously well child awakens suddenly with stridor and coughing, which lasts 45 to 90 minutes before abating spontaneously. It recurs in an irregular pattern. Although steroids have not been shown to be helpful in infectious LTB, they may be beneficial in spasmodic croup. The usual dose of prednisone is 2 mg/kg/day PO.

TABLE 7–15. COMPARISON OF INFECTIOUS UPPER AIRWAY OBSTRUCTIONS

	LTB	Epiglottitis	Bacterial Tracheitis
Age	6 mo–3 yr	2–7 yr	Any
Onset	Gradual	Sudden	Variable
Organism(s)	Parainfluenza	H. influenzae	S. aureus
Voice	Hoarse	Muffled	Muffled
Cough	Barking	Minimal	Productive
Fever	+/−	++++	+++
Dysphagia	−	++++	−
Drooling	−	++++	−

TABLE 7–16. THERAPY FOR INFECTIOUS LTB

At home
  Mist-humidity
  Antipyretics
  Observation

TABLE 7-16. (continued)

In-hospital
   Mist–humidity
   Racemic epinephrine
   Helium and oxygen
   Intubation

Often categorized and discussed with croup, inappropriately so, is pseudomembranous croup or bacterial tracheitis. They are similar only in that the subglottic trachea is the primary location of disease, but bacterial tracheitis resembles epiglottitis much more than LTB in terms of presentation and therapy. This diagnosis should be considered in the child who is getting worse despite therapy. The airway obstruction is due to thick, purulent mucus that cannot be adequately cleared from the trachea. The most likely organisms responsible for bacterial tracheitis are *S. aureus*, streptococcus, and *H. influenzae*. Most children require intubation with frequent suctioning to maintain a patent airway. Despite an appropriate antibiotic regimen to cover the above named organisms, it is often several days before the child can safely be extubated (unlike epiglottitis, in which extubation can often be achieved in 24 to 48 hours).

BRONCHITIS

The diagnosis of bronchitis is difficult to make in pediatrics because definition is lacking. If simple inflammation of the trachea and major divisions of the bronchi constitute pathogenesis, bronchitis would be synonymous with the common cold. Chronic or recurrent bronchitis is also difficult to define, but most authors suggest that a productive cough is a prominent feature and that symptoms persist for a period of weeks or recur regularly. As contrasted with adults, bronchitis in children is caused almost exclusively by viral agents.

Perhaps the most common cause of chronic cough in pediatrics is reactive airways disease, and this is often labeled bronchitis based on the adult diagnostic criteria. As we discover more and more children who have cough as the primary or only manifestation of reactive airways disease, it will be easier to categorize these patients correctly and treat them with bronchodilators rather than antibiotics. Supporting evidence for reactive airways disease includes: negative sputum cultures; presence of common triggers such as exercise, irritants, and viral infections; and a family history of atopy. In the child old enough to cooperate with pulmonary function testing, reactive airways can be documented by inhalation challenge, exercise challenge, or pre- and postbronchodilator testing. In addition to mimicking bronchitis, reactive airways can mimic recurrent "pneumonia," which is really mucus plugging and atelectasis rather than pneumonia.

PERTUSSIS

There are some acquired infections that produce a long-standing productive cough that deserve additional comment. Despite vigorous immunization programs, pertussis continues to be a commonly seen disease in infants and young children. The clinical course is traditionally divided into three phases: coryzal, paroxysmal, and recovery. During the coryzal phase, the disease is indistinguishable from the common cold. It is during this phase that the organism, *Bordetella pertussis*, is most likely to be isolated; this is also prior to the time of being suspicious enough to seek it. The subsequent phase is that of paroxysmal coughing, often interspersed with loud inspiratory "whoops." Coughing may be triggered by feeding, activity, or crying. Unfortunately, this phase can persist for weeks despite appropriate antibiotic therapy with erythromycin. Cultures are likely to be negative during this phase of the illness when the child is likely to be brought to the physician. Nevertheless, the diagnosis can be made using fluorescent antibody to the organism performed on a posterior nasopharyngeal swab. Diagnosis is strongly suggested by a marked lymphocytosis. Treatment includes erythromycin 50 mg/kg/day divided q6h for 14 days.

Improved culture techniques and surveillance programs have

indicated that several other organisms should be considered in the evaluation of paroxysmal cough. Infants may be infected with the same organisms that cause afebrile pneumonia, whereas school-age children with chronic paroxysmal cough often are infected with *M. pneumoniae*. This clinical presentation has been described as the pertussis syndrome regardless of the causative organism. Unfortunately these children may remain symptomatic for weeks or even months despite therapy.

TABLE 7-17. ORGANISMS ASSOCIATED WITH PERTUSSIS SYNDROME

B. pertussis
B. parapertussis
Adenovirus
Chlamydia trachomatis
M. pneumoniae

SINUSITIS

Acute paranasal sinusitis is a more difficult diagnosis to make in children than in adults because the characteristic symptoms are less likely to be present. Furthermore, there is considerable controversy about sensitivity of laboratory methods for documenting this infection. Maxillary or ethmoidal sinusitis usually follows a viral upper respiratory tract infection. Symptoms commonly include cough, nasal discharge, facial pain, and fever. The diagnosis can be confirmed by x-ray, ultrasound, or CT scan; sinus puncture with culture is the definitive diagnostic test, but is infrequently performed due to its invasive nature. The organisms commonly recovered are considered pathogens when isolated from the sinuses, even though they are part of the normal flora in other parts of the respiratory tract. In the immunocompromised host, fungal organisms may be the infecting agents.

Several antibiotics are effective given orally and include amoxicillin, ampicillin, trimethoprim-sulfamethoxazole, and cefaclor.

TABLE 7-18. ACUTE SINUSITIS

Age	Usually >2 years
Symptoms	Cough, nasal discharge, fever, face pain
Organisms	*S. pneumoniae*
	H. influenzae
	Branhamella catarrhalis
Complications	Cavernous sinus thrombosis
	Periorbital cellulitis
	Meningitis
	Maxillary osteomyelitis
	Brain abscess

8

Gastrointestinal Infections

Amebiasis
Campylobacter
Diarrhea and Dehydration
Food Poisoning
Giardiasis
Hepatitis
Pseudomembranous Colitis
Salmonellosis
Shigellosis
Traveler's Diarrhea
Viral Gastroenteritis
Yersinia

AMEBIASIS

Amebiasis is primarily an infection of the colon, which is caused by the protozoan parasite *Entamoeba histolytica*. The organism exists both in trophozoite and cyst forms. Small trophozoites are 10 to 20 μm in diameter and are not associated with invasiveness. Large forms are usually found in the presence of invasive disease and range from 20 to 60 μm in diameter. The presence of ingested RBCs in the endoplasm of a large trophozoite is the most reliable morphologic feature to identify the organism as *E. histolytica*. The cyst form is 10 to 20 μm in diameter and contains 1 to 4 nuclei. Cysts transmit disease and are resistant to drying, cold, and routine chlorination of water.

E. histolytica is more common in the United States than previously suspected. Its prevalence ranges from 1% in Alaska to 10% in southern states. Worldwide, it is more common in tropical and subtropical climates. There are approximately 3500 cases reported each year in the United States; it is estimated that an additional 40% of cases are undetected. Transmission is via the fecal-oral route following ingestion of contaminated water, raw fruit, or vegetables. Insects and flies have also been implicated and there is possible sexual transmission. Poor sanitation and crowding account for reported epidemics. More severe infection is seen in pregnant women and patients who are immunosuppressed or on steroid medications. The disease is more common in the third to fifth decade of life but all ages, including neonates, have been reported.

TABLE 8-1. CLINICAL FORMS OF AMEBIASIS

Asymptomatic carrier
Dysentery
  Pain
  Tenesmus
  Diarrhea with blood and mucus
  Fever
  Abdominal distention
Extraintestinal
  Liver abscess(es)
  Thoracic involvement
  Cerebral abscess
  Cutaneous (perineal)
  Heart and pericardium
  Larynx
  Scapula
  Stomach
  Aorta

Three forms of the disease exist. Asymptomatic carriage of *E. histolytica* is most common. Occasional vague symptoms such as abdominal pain, fatigue, headache, or cough are observed but may not be related to the presence of ameba in the bowel. Incubation ranges from 8 to 95 days. Invasion of the bowel mucosa produces a dysentery picture. Progression of symptoms is usually gradual over 3 to 4 weeks and dysentery may not occur until later in the course. Abdominal pain and tenesmus are the most common symptoms. Infants may have a much more rapid and fulminant course with severe watery diarrhea and hematochezia. Blood is present in the stools in greater than 95% of patients. The leukocyte count is usually elevated with a left shift but eosinophilia is absent.

On proctoscopic examination, superficial ulcers surrounded by normal mucosa are seen along the bowel wall. These ulcerations may then deepen and enlarge with adjacent mucosa becoming hyperemic and friable. Occasionally, granulation tissue without fibrosis (ameboma) forms. Complications of intestinal disease include necrotizing enterocolitis, toxic megacolon, perforation, abscess formation, stricture, and obstruction from amebomas.

Amebae spread to the liver via the portal circulation. Although less frequent than in adults, liver abscesses are the most common extraintestinal form of amebiasis and occur in 1 to 7% of children with invasive disease. This process is more fulminating in children. Hepatic involvement is ten times more common in men than women; there is no difference between genders in prepubescent children. The right lobe of the liver is more commonly involved than the left lobe and abscesses are usually solitary. The fluid has been typically described as a reddish "anchovy paste" but can be white or green. Amebae are found in the walls of the abscess but rarely within fluid. Little inflammatory reaction is evident in the abscess, which explains normal or minimally elevated liver transaminases.

Clinical symptoms of liver abscesses are abdominal pain, fever, and tender hepatomegaly. A nonproductive cough, decreased diaphragmatic excursion, and pleural effusions may be found but jaundice is unusual. Intestinal disease is found in the majority of children with amebic liver abscesses. Laboratory values include a normal or elevated leukocyte count and an invariably elevated sedimentation rate. Normochromic normocytic mild anemia may be present.

Other extraintestinal manifestations of amebiasis are thought to occur via spread from the liver. Extension into the thoracic cavity is the most common and occurs in 10% of patients with liver abscesses.

Diagnosis is usually made by stool examination. If a specimen cannot be processed within 1 hour, then it should be put into a preservative (PVA) (Chap. 6). Identification of *E. histolytica* in the stools can be difficult. A survey of public and private parasitology laboratories reveals that 20% could not identify the trophozoites and 35% could not identify the cysts. The cysts of *E. histolytica* resemble both *E. coli* and other nonpathologic forms of *Entamoeba*. Stained material obtained from mucus or scrapings from the base of an ulcer obtained during proctoscopic examination may also reveal the organism. Numerous serologic tests are available. Most public health facilities use indirect hemagglutination (IHA), which is positive in 58% of asymptomatic patients, 61% of those with moderate involvement, and 95% with severe involvement. A high percentage (close to 100%) of patients with extraintestinal amebiasis have positive antibody titers. Serology is less sensitive in newborns and young infants, even in the presence of severe extraintestinal amebiasis. An elevated titer does not differentiate between acute or past infection and titers may remain positive for 6 months to 3 years after the acute infection. A high titer (greater than or equal to 1:512) is more suggestive of recent infection.

Liver abscesses may be diagnosed by several methods. Technesium sulfur colloid and gallium 67 citrate scans have been used. CT or ultrasonic examination of the abdomen are more sensitive and can be used to follow the size of the abscess.

TABLE 8-2. DIAGNOSIS OF AMEBIASIS

Colonic involvement
  Examination of stool or mucus from bowel
  Biopsy of colonic ulcer
  Serology

TABLE 8-2. (continued)

Hepatic involvement
    Scintography
    CT
    Ultrasound
    Serology

Decisions for therapy and its duration are guided by location and severity of disease.

TABLE 8-3. TREATMENT OF AMEBIASIS

Asymptomatic	Metronidazole 35–50 mg/kg/day PO div q8h × 10 days (maximum 2.4 g/day)
Intestinal	Metronidazole (as above) *PLUS* iodoquinol 40 mg/kg/day PO div q8h × 20 days
Extraintestinal	Same as intestinal *OR* dehydroemetine 1 mg/kg/day IM div q12h × 10 days *PLUS* Chloroquine 10 mg/kg/day PO div q24h × 14 days *PLUS* Iodoquinol (as above)

Most liver abscesses do not require needle aspiration. Drainage is indicated for subcapsular hepatic abscesses or abscesses of the left lobe as these can rupture into the pleural cavity or pericardium. If a liver abscess does not respond to medication, closed needle aspiration under CT or ultrasound guidance may be necessary. If no response is seen, a laparotomy and open drainage should be undertaken. Other indications for surgery are perforation of the bowel with abscess formation if unresponsive to conservative therapy. Brain abscesses should be treated with early drainage through a burr hole and the abscess size followed carefully by CT. If a response is not seen, more definitive surgery may be needed. Pericardial involvement is treated by repeated needle aspirations. Antibiotics are only necessary in patients with secondary infection. Corticosteroids should not be given as this increases the severity of disease.

CAMPYLOBACTER

Campylobacter gastroenteritis has been identified as one of the leading causes of bacterial infection of the gastrointestinal tract in children. The primary organism, which causes disease in children, was formerly termed *Campylobacter fetus* subspecies *jejuni* but is currently referred to as *C. jejuni*.

TABLE 8-4. CLINICAL CHARACTERISTICS OF CAMPYLOBACTER

Incubation period	1–10 days (mean 3–5 days)
Transmission	Contaminated food and water
	Vertical
	Person-to-person (family, day-care centers)
	Animals (chickens, dogs, pigs, cats)
Duration of illness	Mean 7 days, can be recurrent or chronic

The incidence of intrafamilial spread of infection occurs at a much lower rate than would be expected. This probably indicates that the organism is not viable for a long period of time outside the body. Several instances of spread from animals to humans have been recorded and include either direct contact and contamination from the animal or ingestion of contaminated meat that has been inadequately cooked.

Fever, diarrhea, and abdominal pain are the primary symptoms noted. The fever can be quite high and the children may appear toxic. Hematochezia has been found to be present in at least half the children and typically appears several days after the onset of the illness. Abdominal pain may be so severe as to suggest an acute abdomen. Many patients complain of malaise and fatigue. These are especially prominent in the recurrent form of the illness and may be the only symptoms present between bouts of diarrhea. Vomiting is noted in approximately one-third of patients but is usually mild and does not result in dehydration.

TABLE 8-5. SYMPTOMS OF CAMPYLOBACTER INFECTION

Fever
Diarrhea
Hematochezia
Abdominal pain
Malaise
Vomiting
Toxic appearance

There are several presentations of campylobacter gastroenteritis with the most common form being self-limited diarrhea lasting up to 1 week. Recurrent or chronic diarrhea can occur and campylobacter has been implicated as a cause of traveler's diarrhea. Campylobacter can cause an exacerbation of symptoms in patients with previously diagnosed inflammatory bowel disease resembling a relapse of their primary disease. Involvement of the gut can also result in toxic megacolon. Concomitant infection with salmonella, shigella, giardia, and rotavirus has been documented.

TABLE 8-6. GI MANIFESTATIONS OF CAMPYLOBACTER

Recurrent or chronic diarrhea
Traveler's diarrhea
Colitis or enterocolitis
   Ulcerative
   Nodular (Crohn's-like)
   Pseudomembranous
Massive GI bleeding

(*continued*)

TABLE 8-6. (continued)

Acute abdomen
    Cholecystitis
    Pancreatitis
    Appendicitis
    Mesenteric lymphadenitis
Exacerbation of inflammatory bowel disease
Toxic megacolon

The most common extraintestinal manifestation of campylobacter is reactive arthritis occurring more frequently in men with
the HLA-B27 histocompatibility antigen.

TABLE 8-7. EXTRAINTESTINAL MANIFESTATIONS OF CAMPYLOBACTER

Reiter's syndrome
Reactive arthritis
Septic arthritis
Meningitis
Bacteremia
UTI
Glomerulonephritis
Carditis

The diagnosis of campylobacter by stool culture is relatively
easy with selective medium. Direct examination of the stool is
usually positive for RBCs and leukocytes. Dark field or phase
contrast microscopic examination reveals the characteristic dart-
ing motion of the *C. jejuni* organism. A recently described technique for staining of the stool smear with fuchsin has been shown
to have a good correlation with stool cultures. This technique
lends itself to the office setting and has proven useful for early
detection of campylobacter infections.

Treatment may not be necessary in children with mild disease. Many patients are asymptomatic when the diagnosis by stool culture is made. With treatment, stool cultures become negative within 72 hours; with no treatment campylobacter can be cultured from stool for up to several weeks. The incidence of intrafamilial spread of campylobacter is low and spread of disease from asymptomatic excreters has not been documented. If treatment is initiated, erythromycin is the drug of choice. The oral dosage is 40 to 50 mg/kg/day divided q6h for 7 to 10 days. For systemic infection, gentamicin may be added or substituted. Parenteral therapy is probably not needed for asymptomatic bacteremia.

TABLE 8-8. TREATMENT OF CAMPYLOBACTER[a]

Enteritis
Erythromycin
Systemic
Gentamicin
Erythromycin or chloramphenicol
Alternatives
Tetracycline
Doxycycline or clindamycin

[a] For dosages see Tables 18-12 and 18-13.

DIARRHEA AND DEHYDRATION

One of the most common diseases encountered in pediatrics is gastroenteritis. Most episodes are mild and self-limited. The child is particularly vulnerable to dehydration as a consequence of diarrhea, however, and this may result in the need for hospitalization for rehydration and correction of acid-base or electrolyte disturbances. Acute infectious diarrheal illnesses may be caused by bacteria, viruses, or protozoa.

Some of the more common causes of acute infectious diarrhea may be differentiated on clinical grounds.

TABLE 8-9. COMPARISON OF CLINICAL FINDINGS IN ACUTE INFECTIOUS DIARRHEA

	Shigella	Salmonella	Campylobacter	Rotavirus
Vomiting	Rare	Common	±	Common
Fever	Present	Variable	Present	Variable
Stool volume	Small	Moderate	Moderate	Large
Stool consistency	Viscous	Slimy	Watery	Watery
Stool odor	Odorless	Foul	Foul	Odorless
Stool blood	++++	Variable	Common	±
Stool mucus	++++	Moderate	Variable	Absent
Stool WBCs	++++	++++	Present	±
Bronchitis	Common	Absent	±	±

Treatment of diarrhea is predominantly supportive with correction of fluid and electrolyte abnormalites. Antibiotic therapy is recommended in some forms of bacterial or protozoan diarrhea (see individual sections).

Treatment of dehydration requires recognition of the type of dehydration present, as well as its severity.

TABLE 8-10. COMPARISON OF TYPES OF DEHYDRATION

	Isonatremic Dehydration	Hyponatremic Dehydration	Hypernatremic Dehydration
Sodium and water deficit	Proportionate loss of water and sodium	Loss of sodium in excess of water	Loss of water in excess of sodium

TABLE 8-10. (continued)

	Isonatremic Dehydration	Hyponatremic Dehydration	Hypernatremic Dehydration
Serum sodium	Normal	<130	>150
Frequency of occurrence in diarrhea	70%	10%	20%
Clinical setting commonly seen	Any diarrhea	Diarrhea with cholera-type stools and/or replacement with free water	Diarrheal losses replaced with fluid of high salt content
Extracellular fluid volume	↓↓	↓↓↓	↓
Intracellular fluid volume	Normal	↑	↓

Because of the relative preservation of extracellular fluid volume in hypernatremic dehydration and the greater depletion of extracellular fluid volume in hyponatremic dehydration compared with isotonic dehydration, modifications must be made accordingly in the assessment by physical examination.

TABLE 8-11. ESTIMATION OF VOLUME DEFICIT FROM PHYSICAL EXAMINATION

	Isonatremic		
	5%	10%	15%
	Hyponatremic		
	<5%	5%	10%
	Hypernatremic		
	10%	15%	>15%
Level of consciousness[a]	Normal or lethargic	Obtunded or stuporous	Comatose
Mucous membranes	Dry	Dry	Parched
Skin turgor	Fair	Poor	Very poor

(continued)

TABLE 8-11. (continued)

Eyes	Normal	Absence of tears	Sunken
Perfusion	Normal	Decreased	Shock

[a] Level of consciousness may be more affected in hypernatremic dehydration.

The extracellular volume deficit may be estimated from the formula:

$$\text{Volume (ml)} = \% \text{ dehydration} \times \text{weight (kg)} \times 10.$$

The sodium deficit in hyponatremic dehydration may be estimated from the formula:

$$\text{Na(mEq)} = (140 - \text{serum sodium}) \times 0.6 \times \text{weight (kg)}.$$

TABLE 8-12. TREATMENT OF DEHYDRATION

Isonatremic dehydration

Fluid resuscitation for shock	Volume: 40 ml/kg over 20-30 min; repeat as necessary to achieve hemodynamic stability or until CVP ≥ 10 mm Hg or PCWP ≥ 12 mm Hg Fluid: Isotonic crystalloid solution (Ringer's lactate or normal saline)
First 24 hr	Volume: Replace deficit over 6-8 hr (less amount infused during fluid resuscitation phase) *PLUS* maintenance fluid requirement for 24 hr *PLUS* any abnormal ongoing losses as they occur Fluid: 5–10% dextrose with Na 75 mEq/L, Cl 55 mEq/L, and bicarbonate, lactate, or acetate 20 mEq/L

TABLE 8-12. (continued)

Hypernatremic dehydration
  Fluid resuscitation for shock — Volume: 20 ml/kg over 20–30 min; repeat as necessary to achieve hemodynamic stability or until CVP $\geq$ 12 mm Hg
  Fluid: 5% albumin or Plasmanate

  First 24 hr — Volume: Replace deficit over 48 hr (less amount infused during fluid resuscitation phase) *PLUS* maintenance fluid requirement for 48 hr *PLUS* any abnormal ongoing losses as they occur
  Fluid: 5% dextrose with Na 35 mEq/L, Cl 20 mEq/L, and lactate or acetate 15 mEq/L
  Calcium: Add 1 amp of 10% calcium gluconate to first 500 ml IV fluids
  Potassium: Add K 40 mEq/L as soon as urine flow has resumed

Hyponatremic dehydration
  Fluid resuscitation for shock — Volume: 20 ml/kg over 20–30 min; repeat as necessary to achieve hemodynamic stability or until CVP $\geq$ 10 mm Hg or PCWP $\geq$ 12 mm Hg
  Fluid: 5% albumin or Plasmanate

  First 24 hr — Volume: Replace 2/3 of deficit over first 24 hr *PLUS* maintenance fluid requirement for 24 hr *PLUS* any abnormal ongoing losses as they occur
  Fluid: 5% dextrose with Na 75 mEq/L *PLUS* 2/3 of calculated Na deficit in first 24 hr fluids. Proportion of anion as Cl vs. bicarbonate, lactate, or acetate to be determined by degree of metabolic acidosis present

  Second 24 hr — Volume: Replace remaining 1/3 of deficit over second 24 hr *PLUS* maintenance fluid requirement for 24 hr *PLUS* any
(continued)

TABLE 8-12. (continued)

abnormal ongoing losses as they
occur
Fluid: 5% dextrose with Na 75
mEq/L *PLUS* 1/3 of calculated
Na deficit in second 24 hr fluids.
Proportion of anion as Cl vs.
bicarbonate, lactate, or acetate to
be determined by degree of
metabolic acidosis present
Potassium: Begin replacement of
3 mEq/kg/day during second
24 hr

The neurologic symptoms in hypernatremic dehydration may
be even more pronounced. When the hypernatremic state develops, the brain cells protect their intracellular volume to a certain
extent from loss of water by generation of idiogenic osmoles. It is
not known, however, how rapidly these osmoles can develop nor
the speed with which they again disappear when the hypernatremic state is corrected. The adequacy of this protective mechanism
may determine the extent of neurologic sequelae such as seizures
or permanent brain damage. It is not uncommon for seizures to
occur during the course of treatment for dehydration.

TABLE 8-13. TREATMENT OF SEIZURES ASSOCIATED WITH DEHYDRATION

Dehydration	Causes of Seizures	Treatment
Hyponatremic	Water intoxication	Correction of low serum Na up to 125 mEq/L: 3 mEq/kg NaCl (as 3% NaCl or Na quadrate 4 mEq/ml) IV over 3 min; repeat prn until seizures stop (not to exceed 15 mEq/kg)

TABLE 8-13. (continued)

Dehydration	Causes of Seizures	Treatment
Hypernatremic	Cerebral intracellular water shift during rehydration; most likely to occur with drop in serum Na faster than 10 mEq/L/24 hr	Mannitol 20%, 0.25 g/kg IV over 15 min

FOOD POISONING

Bacterial food poisoning may be caused by a variety of organisms with the most common being *Salmonella* and *Staphylococcus aureus*. At least 300 outbreaks of food-borne disease are reported each year with this likely being 10 to 100 times an underestimation of episodes. The majority of patients experience self-limited disease. Disease may be produced by ingestion of preformed toxin, elaboration of toxin into the gastrointestinal tract, or direct invasion of mucosa by organisms. Ingestion of preformed toxin is associated with a shorter incubation period. Most patients will require only supportive therapy. The major exception is botulism which represents a medical emergency (see Chap. 1).

TABLE 8-14. EPIDEMIOLOGIC AND CLINICAL ASPECTS OF FOOD POISONING

Organism	Pathogenesis	Source	Prevention
Salmonella	Infection	Meats, poultry, dairy products	Proper cooking and food handling
Staphylococcus	Preformed enterotoxin	Meats, fowl, potato salad, cream-filled pastry, cheese, sausage	Careful food handling and rapid refrigeration
Clostridium perfringens	Enterotoxin	Meats, poultry	Avoid delay in serving foods, avoid cooling and rewarming foods
C. botulism	Preformed neurotoxin	Home canned goods, uncooked	Proper refrigeration
Vibrio parahaemolyticus	Infection enterotoxin	Seafish, seawater, shellfish	Proper refrigeration
Bacillus cereus Vomiting type	Preformed toxin	Cooked rice, vegetables, meats, cereal, pudding	Proper refrigeration of cooked rice and other foods
Diarrhea type	Unproven		

Organism	Incubation	Symptoms	Duration	Treatment
Salmonella	8–72 hr average 12–18 hr	Diarrhea (blood), abdominal pain, fever, chills, nausea, vomiting	3–5 days	None unless severe

Organism	Incubation period	Symptoms	Duration/Outcome	Treatment
Staphylococcus	1–6 hr	Severe vomiting, abdominal pain, diarrhea	6–8 hr	None
C. perfringens	8–24 hr average 8–12 hr	Watery diarrhea, crampy abdominal pain, nausea, vomiting rare	≤ 24 hr	None
C. botulism	12–36 hr	Nausea, vomiting, diarrhea, dysphagia, dysarthria muscle weakness, respiratory paralysis	Death within several days unless treated	Supportive (see Chap. 1)
V. parahaemolyticus	4–48 hr 13–24 hr average	Severe watery diarrhea, abdominal cramps, nausea and vomiting, fever, chills, can produce dysentery	2 hr–10 days	None
B. cereus				
Vomiting type	1–6 hr	Vomiting, abdominal pain	8–24 hr	None
Diarrhea type	6–12 hr	Diarrhea, abdominal pain, vomiting	20–36 hr	None

GIARDIASIS

Giardia lamblia is second only to *Enterobius vermicularis* (pinworm) as the most common parasite found in the United States and is a major pathogen in children. Giardiasis is especially prevalent in day-care centers, institutional care facilities, areas with overcrowding, and in the tropics. Children are more often affected than adults with person-to-person being the most common route of transmission. Infants and toddlers may be an important reservoir as up to 50% are asymptomatic. Prevalence rates in day-care centers range from 17 to 90% with an average of 20 to 30%. Originally persons with achlorhydria or hypogammaglobulinemia were thought to be more susceptible to infection; however, the incidence of giardiasis in these populations is not different from the general population.

Clinical symptoms vary with age; younger children are more likely to be symptomatic.

TABLE 8–15. GIARDIASIS: CLINICAL SYMPTOMS

No symptoms
Diarrhea
Weight loss, failure to thrive
Anorexia
Vomiting
Abdominal cramps
Constipation
Malodorous stools

Diagnosis of giardiasis is best achieved by examination of three stool samples by a laboratory with expertise in parasitology. Detection of trophozoites requires examination of fresh stools but as the majority of children do not pass trophozoites, examination of a recently passed stool is not necessary for diagnosis. Cysts are quite hardy and will keep at room temperature; however, because infection with more than one parasite is frequently encountered, fixatives to preserve both trophozoites and cysts allow detection of other parasites. These also have the convenience of home collection of samples as the bottles containing fixatives can be mailed to the laboratory. Although the detection rate of *Giardia* cysts can be as high as 97% with three stool samples, other methods for diagnosis are available.

TABLE 8-16. GIARDIASIS: DIAGNOSIS

Stool examination—fresh or with fixatives
Duodenal fluid examination
    Entero-Test capsule[a]
    Intubation of small bowel
Biopsy of duodenum or jejunum
Serology
CIE of stool

[a] Health Development Corporation, Palo Alto, Calif.

Three medications are currently used for treatment of infection. The major advantage of furazolidone is the liquid dosage form. Atabrine has had extensive use, is less expensive but not as well tolerated by children. Metronidazole has proven to be effective but is expensive and not approved for the treatment of giardiasis in children. All of these medications produce an antabuse-like effect and medications containing alcohol should not be given concomitantly. Persistent symptoms after therapy may indicate small bowel overgrowth or incomplete eradication of the pathogen requiring a second course of medication.

TABLE 8-17. TREATMENT OF GIARDIASIS

	Furazolidone	Quinacrine	Metronidazole
Advantages	Liquid form Few side effects	High cure rate Experience Inexpensive	High cure rate Availability

(continued)

TABLE 8-17. (continued)

	Furazolidone	Quinacrine	Metronidazole
Disadvantages	Lower cure rate	Bitter taste	Not approved
		Side effects	Expensive
	Longer duration of therapy	Tablet form only	Tablet form only
	Large volume of liquid for preschool age		Mutagenic/ carcinogenic in animals
Dosage (mg/kg/day)	8	6	15
Schedule	q6h × 10 days	q8h × 7 days	q8h × 7 days
Dosage form	100 mg tab	10 mg tab	250 mg tab
	50 mg/15ml susp		500 mg tab

HEPATITIS

The clinical presentation of jaundice following a prodrome of anorexia, nausea, vomiting, and right upper quadrant pain suggests a diagnosis of hepatitis and dictates a serologic evaluation for etiology. Most cases are caused by the viruses hepatitis A (HAV) or hepatitis B (HB). Other agents should be considered when screening for HAV and HB is negative. Hepatitis is often asymptomatic in children, particularly HAV in infants less than 18 months of age.

TABLE 8-18. DIFFERENTIAL ETIOLOGY OF HEPATITIS

HAV
HBV
Non-A, non-B viral hepatitis
EBV
CMV
Leptospirosis
Noninfectious
   Drug induced (INH, erythromycin)
   Obstructive jaundice

Etiologic diagnosis is made by serologic evaluation and should be accomplished rapidly so that decisions for prophylactic administration of gammaglobulin (for HAV) or hyperimmune HB immune globulin to family members might be made (see Chap. 3). If a delay in laboratory testing is anticipated, family members should receive gammaglobulin (0.02 ml/kg, maximum 2 ml) because this is inexpensive and must be given early to protect against HAV.

Therapy for patients with HAV or HBV is supportive and most can be managed at home. Indications for hospital admission include intractable vomiting, an elevated prothrombin time, and impending hepatic coma.

Those with HAV are contagious for 2 weeks after the onset of jaundice whereas individuals with HB are infective while they are seropositive for HB surface antigen (HB_s Ag) or have anti-HB core antibody (anti-HB_c) but lack antibody to surface antigen (anti-HB_s). While contagious, patients should be advised as to stool and blood precautions and sexual transmission of disease. Only HB is associated with a chronic carrier state.

TABLE 8-19. SEROLOGIC DIAGNOSIS OF HAV AND HBV

Initial screen
  Anti-HAV IgM
  HB_s Ag
  Anti-HB_c IgM
Follow-up monitoring for HB (at 1 mo and q3mo as indicated)
  HB_s Ag
  Anti-HB_c
  Anti-HB_s

Recommendations for HB vaccine in high-risk groups are reviewed in Chapter 3.

PSEUDOMEMBRANOUS COLITIS (PMC)

PMC is an inflammatory condition in the colon, which is associated with antibiotic use. The etiology has been determined to be *Clostridium difficile* toxin.

Virtually all antibiotics have been associated with PMC. In children, more cases have been reported following administration of ampicillin but this simply reflects the widespread use of this antibiotic. The route, dose, and length of treatment for the antibiotic are not related to the development of PMC.

The diarrhea associated with PMC is usually of rapid onset and the patient may experience 10 to 20 stools a day, although children tend to have less severe diarrhea. At least half of patients have blood and/or fecal leukocytes in the stool. Abdominal pain and tenderness can occur although they are not predominant symptoms. The tenderness can be so severe as to mimic an acute abdomen. Fever, anorexia, nausea, and vomiting are part of the symptom complex.

The onset of disease is usually within 4 to 10 days of initiation of antibiotics. It has been seen within 4 hours of initiation and as long as 6 weeks after. At least one-third of the patients have the onset of disease after the antibiotics have been stopped. The exact incidence of PMC is not known, but appears to be less common in children than in adults.

As demonstration of disease is within reach of the rigid proctoscope in the majority of patients, rigid proctosigmoidoscopy is the preferred method of diagnosis. Flexible sigmoidoscopy, which reaches to 60 cm is an alternative. Both are inexpensive procedures and can be readily performed as outpatients, even in children. The demonstration of *C. difficile* toxin in the stool is of importance in confirming the diagnosis. Toxin is present in 97 to 100% of patients with endoscopic evidence for PMC. Approximately one-fourth of children with antibiotic-associated diarrhea but no colitis, however, also have toxin in their stools. Stool cultures are of little diagnostic use because asymptomatic colonization with this organism is common, particularly in neonates and infants.

General supportive care and fluids are important aspects of

treatment. Antiperistaltic medication should not be used as they may prolong colonization with *C. difficile*. If the patient is hospitalized, simple isolation or enteric precautions should be observed. There is some controversy concerning the need to discontinue the offending antibiotic. Drugs used in the therapy of PMC are efficacious if used concurrently with the offending antibiotic. Most investigators favor discontinuation of the initial antibiotic.

TABLE 8-20. TREATMENT OF PMC

Fluids, supportive care
Avoidance of antiperistaltic medications
Discontinue offending antibiotic
Simple isolation
Vancomycin 50 mg/kg (maximum 2 g) PO div q8h or metronidazole 25 mg/kg PO div q6h × 7-14 days

The relapse rate is 12 to 20% and usually begins 4 to 20 days after the initial treatment. Clinically, the patients experience the same symptoms and signs as during their initial bout of PMC. *C. difficile* and the toxin can again be isolated, even though during the period between initial treatment and relapse these two may not have been detected. Patients who have diverticulitis or who are granulocytopenic are more likely to relapse. The ability of the organism to undergo sporolation is probably the most important factor in relapse. The spore form is rather insensitive to antibiotics and therefore may not be eradicated with treatment. Reinfection from the environment is also a possibility as *C. difficile* can readily be cultured in the room of patients hospitalized for PMC. It also can be found in their home environment and on the hands of hospital personnel. *C. difficile* inoculated into a carpet can be recovered for up to 5 months and is resistant to many routine cleaners.

The treatment for relapse has not been established in children; however, in adults a second course of vancomycin at the original dosage is recommended for 2 to 3 weeks.

SALMONELLOSIS

Salmonella sp. are common pathogens causing bacterial gastroenteritis in children. Although there are over 2000 serotypes, 10 account for approximately two-thirds of total isolates. Clinically, salmonella organisms are divided into those strains that cause enteric fever such as *S. typhi*, *S. paratyphi* A, *S. paratyphi* B, and *S. cholerae-suis*, and those more commonly associated with other forms of disease.

TABLE 8–21. CLINICAL FORMS OF SALMONELLOSIS

Gastroenteritis
Enteric fever
Bacteremia
Localized infection
Chronic carrier

Gastroenteritis is the most common form and accounts for most of the salmonella infections in the United States. In other countries enteric fever is more common as *S. typhi* is the predominant species. Bacteremia tends to occur in the young and the old with approximately 40% of cases being present in children less than 5 years of age. Neonates accounted for the highest percentage of this group; however, breast feeding provides protection against salmonellosis. Localized infections are frequently due to *S. cholerae-suis*.

TABLE 8–22. FOCAL INFECTIONS OF SALMONELLA

Meningitis	Cholecystitis
Brain abscess and empyema	Salpingitis
Endocarditis	UTI
Pericarditis	Osteomyelitis
Mycotic aneurysm	Arthritis
	Myocardial abscess

TABLE 8-22. (continued)

Necrotizing enterocolitis	Reiter's syndrome
Appendicitis	Pneumonia and empyema
Abdominal abscess	Endophthalmitis

A chronic carrier state can also be established. This more often occurs following enteric fever in patients with gallbladder disease. One study demonstrated that a chronic carrier state (defined by excretion greater than 1 year) was seen in 2.6% of patients who were infected with nontyphi salmonella. Most chronic carriers were less than 5 years of age.

TABLE 8-23. CHARACTERISTICS OF SALMONELLA GASTROENTERITIS

Incubation	8–72 hr (mean 12–48 hr)
Season	Warm weather
Peak age	1–6 mo
Transmission	Food, animals, marijuana, fomite, flies, insects, person-to-person
Site of involvement	Distal small bowel, colon
Duration of symptoms	2–7 days

Salmonella may be introduced by a food handler or processor. It is resistant to mild refrigeration, and thus, undercooked food is a potential source of contamination and transmission of the disease in major outbreaks.

Symptoms can begin quite abruptly. The distal small bowel and colon are the predominant sites of involvement. Salmonellae invade the lamina propria, which induces an inflammatory reaction and release of prostaglandins. Prostaglandin release stimulates cyclic AMP, which in itself causes secretory diarrhea. An endotoxin can be isolated but may not be active in the pathogenesis of the disease. The damage to the cell is not as extensive as with shigella, and thus, the colitis and enteritis are not as destructive. Because the organism is limited to the upper layers of the gut mucosa, normal mechanisms of elimination allow clearance of salmonella in a rapid manner.

TABLE 8-24. SYMPTOMS AND LABORATORY FINDINGS IN SALMONELLA GASTROENTERITIS

Symptoms
   Diarrhea
   Fever >102F
   Abdominal pain
   Distended abdomen
   Vomiting
   Constitutional symptoms
   Tenesmus
   Hematochezia
Laboratory findings
   Elevated WBC count
   Guaiac positive stool
   PMNs on stool smears (85%)
   Positive stool culture

Salmonella gastroenteritis is, in general, a self-limited disease; however, there are several conditions that may influence its ability to cause sepsis or other complications.

TABLE 8-25. FACTORS AFFECTING INFECTION

Age <12 mo
Decreased gastric acidity
Stress—cold, malnutrition
Antibiotics
Depressed immune function
Hemolysis

Neonates and infants less than 3 months of age are more prone to sepsis and meningitis than other age groups. Patients with sickle cell anemia have a higher incidence of osteomyelitis due to salmonella. The ability to cause extraintestinal and focal infections with salmonella is partly dependent upon the state of the host, the species of salmonella involved, and the inoculum dose.

Although gastroenteritis or localized infections are by far the most common forms of salmonella, enteric fever still occurs in the United States. The term typhoid fever has been mostly abandoned since organisms other than *S. typhi* can cause an identical picture.

TABLE 8-26. ENTERIC FEVER

Organism	*S. typhi*, paratyphoid strains
Transmission	Human reservoir, contaminated food or water, insect vectors
Season	All
Incubation	3–56 days (mean, 10 days)
Symptoms	Fever, headache, chills, diarrhea, vomiting, abdominal pain, cough
Signs	Rose spots, hepatosplenomegaly, neurologic signs, relative bradycardia

S. typhi is somewhat unique in that there is no natural host in nature other than humans. The main route of spread of disease is by food or water that has been contaminated by human fecal material. There are some instances of possible transmission by insect vectors; however, this has not been absolutely established.

There are four phases of the disease. The first phase is a flu-like illness, during which time the patient may also have symptoms of gastroenteritis. The second phase demonstrates the multisystem invasion by the organism. Patients show encephalopathic changes, bronchitis, and evidence of reticuloendothelial system involvement with hepatosplenomegaly and lymphadenopathy. Relative bradycardia usually occurs during this period, which begins approximately 2 to 3 weeks after ingestion of the organism. High fever can be seen and without treatment can persist for 2 to 3 weeks. Because of GI involvement, perforation or hemorrhage is a risk. If the disease does not abate, a third phase is entered during which metastatic phenomena such as myocarditis occur. The last phase is the carrier state, which occurs in approximately 3% of patients. The presence of gallbladder disease markedly enhances the chances of becoming a chronic carrier. Chronic carriage is more common in adult women, but this may be related to the fact that gallbladder disease is more common in this group.

Diagnosis of enteric fever is made on clinical grounds, serologic (salmonella O and H antibody) measurement, and with cultures. During the initial stages of enteric fever, stool cultures may be positive; however, there is an increasing yield from the stool culture during the third and fourth week of disease. Initially, blood cultures are negative but once the disease is established the blood cultures can be positive in 80 to 90% of the patients. Other sites, which can be cultured, are bone marrow and biopsy of rose spots. Antibody titers (febrile agglutinins) become positive after the first week of illness.

Salmonella gastroenteritis is usually not treated, as antibiotics simply prolong the carrier state. There are specific instances when treatment is indicated. These include patients who are more prone to have invasive disease or already have established severe disease.

TABLE 8-27. INDICATIONS FOR TREATMENT OF SALMONELLA GASTROENTERITIS

Infants <3 mo of age
Toxic or severe disease
Immunodeficiency
Malignancy

Ampicillin, amoxicillin, chloramphenicol, and TMP-SMX are all effective for susceptible organisms. Ampicillin is the usual drug of choice but selection is dependent on local sensitivities.

Detection of salmonella in stool cultures following therapy does not necessitate a second course of treatment.

TABLE 8-28. TREATMENT OF SALMONELLOSIS

	Drug	Daily Dose (mg/kg)	Duration (days)
Gastroenteritis (if indicated)	Ampicillin	100	7
	TMP–SMX	10–50	7
		(either PO or IV)	
Localized or focal infection	As directed by process and location		
Enteric fever	Chloramphenicol	50–100	14
	Ampicillin	100–200	14
	TMP–SMX	20–100	14
		(usually IV)	
Bacteremia	Same as enteric fever		10–12
Chronic carrier	No dosage established in children		

The local public health department should be notified of all cases of salmonella infection because this is a reportable disease.

SHIGELLOSIS

Shigella is a nonmotile gram-negative rod. There are 39 serotypes divided into four groups: group A, *Shigella dysenteriae*; group B, *S. flexneri*; group C, *S. boydii*; and group D, *S. sonnei*. In the United States and many developed nations *S. sonnei* is responsible for the majority of GI infections. Virulence of these organisms is related to the presence of a complex antigen side chain to the envelope that allows the organism to invade the gastrointestinal cell. Virulent organisms are termed "smooth" where avirulent organisms are termed "rough." The toxin of *S. dysenteriae* has been the most intensely studied. It is known to be an exotoxin and neurotoxin and produces transudation of fluid in ileal loops of experimental animals. It is also a cytotoxin that can induce cell death by suppression of cell protein synthesis. There is mounting evidence that similar toxins are also produced by the other virulent strains of *Shigella*. In order for the organism to produce disease it must attach to the cell wall and invade the cell. The organism then multiplies and spreads to adjacent cells. Toxins may aid in the spread.

Transmission of disease occurs via the oral/anal route.

TABLE 8-29. SHIGELLA GASTROENTERITIS

Transmission	Food, water, houseflies
Incubation	1–3 days
Duration of illness	3–7 days
Season	Increased in winter
Age	Less than 10 yr, peak incidence 2 yr old

Contaminated food and water are the primary sources associated with epidemics of shigellosis; however, houseflies may also transmit disease. *Shigella* can be cultured from toilet seats for up to 17 days postinoculation. There may be asymptomatic carriers that contribute to spread of the disease and *Shigella* may survive in food for up to 30 days. Unlike other enteric pathogens, a very small number of organisms (200) is needed to produce disease.

The incubation period of *Shigella* is 1 to 3 days and the duration of illness in an uncomplicated case is 3 to 7 days. There is an increased incidence during the winter months. The majority of patients are less than 10 years of age with a peak incidence at 2 years of age.

In children the diarrhea is watery and voluminous with blood in the stools usually noted 24 to 48 hours after initial symptoms. The stool volume may then decrease, with a frequent stooling pattern. Respiratory symptoms and fever are prominent features.

Proctoscopic examination reveals intense inflammation with crypt abscesses. If severe dysentery is present a pseudomembrane can be seen.

TABLE 8-30. DIAGNOSIS OF SHIGELLA INFECTION

Stool smear for WBCs
Stool culture
Presence of leukocytosis
Increased absolute band count (more bands than PMNs)

There are several culture media that will support the growth of *Shigella*; stool specimens should be plated as soon as possible to achieve the best results. The stool smear typically shows a large amount of WBCs with predominant PMNs and bands. Leukocytosis is also seen with the band count greater than the neutrophil count in 32 to 85% of patients. A high absolute band count is also seen with *Campylobacter* and *Salmonella*.

There are many complications of shigellosis; however, the majority of the complications are associated with *S. dysenteriae*. Dehydration can be seen with any of the *Shigella* species.

TABLE 8-31. COMPLICATIONS OF SHIGELLOSIS

Dehydration
Bacteremia-sepsis
Intestinal perforation
Rectal prolapse
Hemolytic-uremic syndrome
Reiter's syndrome
Eye involvement
UTI
Pneumonia
Seizures (neurotoxin)

The incidence of bacteremia and sepsis with shigellosis ranges from 0.6 to 7%. The majority of children are less than 5 years of age and there is a 35 to 50% mortality with bacteremia. Children with bacteremia more frequently present with dehydration, afebrile, and with malnutrition. The majority of them are also malnourished. Blood cultures are most often positive during the first and second day of the disease.

Another common complication is seizures associated with all species of *Shigella*. The incidence varies from 10 to 45% in children up to 7 years of age. The mechanism for the seizure may be related to the fever or a neurotoxin; however, the etiology is not definitively established.

There is presently a high incidence of ampicillin resistance among isolates of *Shigella*. Drug selection therefore depends on local sensitivities to ampicillin and TMP-SMX.

TABLE 8–32. THERAPY FOR SHIGELLOSIS

TMP-SMX	5–10 mg/25–50 mg/kg/day div bid for 5 days
	OR
Ampicillin	100 mg/kg/day div qid for 5 days

Fever should defervesce in 12 to 20 hours with therapy and improvement in the diarrhea should be seen in 1 to 3 days. *Shigella* is eliminated within the first and second day after initiation of therapy. If therapy is not instituted, it can be cultured from stool for up to 1 month. This may influence the decision to treat children with mild enteritis. Antidiarrheal drugs should be discouraged as they prolong the fever, diarrhea, and excretion of the organism.

The mortality of uncomplicated gastroenteritis is less than 1%. Chronic carriage of the organism in the stool is very unusual unless the patient was initially malnourished.

TRAVELER'S DIARRHEA

Traveler's diarrhea affects 25 to 50% of people who visit foreign countries. Numerous organisms are responsible with the vast majority being due to enterotoxigenic *Escherichia coli* (ETEC) in Americans who travel to Mexico or South America. Giardia is a more likely pathogen for travelers to the Soviet Union.

TABLE 8-33. ETIOLOGY OF TRAVELER'S DIARRHEA

Agent	Incidence (%)
ETEC	40–70
Shigella	15–20
Salmonella	10–15
Rotavirus	4–10
Giardia	2–3
E. histolytica	2–3
Undiagnosed	10–30
Others: invasive *E. coli*; *Campylobacter*, *Vibrio parahaemolyticus*	2–3

If meticulous attention is paid to avoiding potentially contaminated food and water, the incidence of infection is extremely low. Prophylactic antibiotics are no longer recommended because their routine use leads to the rapid development of bacterial resistance. Antimicrobial therapy should be reserved for symptomatic cases or for individuals entering an extremely high risk area (poor sanitation) and who will be remaining there for more than 5 days. Recommended antibiotics are trimethoprim-sulfamethoxazole or doxycycline for 5 days (see Table 18-13 for dosages). It is most practical to allow travelers to bring appropriate medication with them if they are staying for more than 5 days, but with instructions to begin therapy only if symptoms occur. Antimotility medications should not be used.

VIRAL GASTROENTERITIS

Viral gastroenteritis is one of the most common illnesses in childhood with a number of etiologic agents identified in sporadic and epidemic cases. The vast majority are due to rotavirus or Norwalk agent, however.

TABLE 8–34. VIRAL ETIOLOGY OF GASTROENTERITIS

Rotavirus
Norwalk agent
Corona virus
Enteroviruses
Astrovirus
Adenovirus
Minirotavirus
Calicivirus

Rotavirus is most common in infants, accounting for one-half of all cases, whereas the Norwalk agent is associated with epidemic disease in school-aged children. Both are transmitted by the fecal-oral route.

TABLE 8–35. CLINICAL ASPECTS OF ROTAVIRUS AND NORWALK AGENT GASTROENTERITIS

	Rotavirus	Norwalk Agent
Incubation	48–72 hr	18–48 hr
Duration of illness	5–8 days	1–2 days
Season	Winter	All
Usual age	6–24 mo	5–10 yr
Diagnosis	Rotazyme	No test available

Treatment is supportive with particular attention focused on the potential development of dehydration (see the Diarrhea and Dehydration section in this chapter).

YERSINIA

Yersinia enterocolitica is a small gram-negative aerobic coccoba-cillus that is responsible for large numbers of cases of gastroen-teritis in Europe and Canada. There are 35 serotypes and 5 biotypes. Some appear primarily to be animal strains. Serotypes 0:3 and 0:9 are most common in human infections in Europe, 0:3 is most common in Canada and 0:8 in the United States. Al-though *Y. enterocolitica* can be isolated from many sources in-cluding wild and domestic animals, milk, water supplies, oysters, and many other foods, the mode of transmission in sporadic cases is unclear. In epidemic cases person-to-person transmission in families or hospitals, and food-borne transmission have been identified. The incubation period is 4 to 10 days.

Clinically, there are several disease forms that seem to be age-related (Table 8–36). Younger children have a milder form of disease with diarrhea being the predominant symptom. They can also have abdominal pain, which may increase and mimic appen-dicitis. The picture of "pseudoappendicitis" is usually seen in older children and adults. This is actually acute mesenteric adeni-tis. Older adolescents and young adults may also have the symp-toms of an acute enteritis with localization of the disease in the area of the terminal ileum. This form of the disease may often be confused with Crohn's disease.

TABLE 8-36. CLINICAL SYNDROMES OF *YERSINIA ENTEROCOLITICA*

Acute diarrhea
  Age: ≤ 5 yr
  Symptoms: diarrhea with or without blood, fever, vomiting
  Duration: 2 wk
Acute mesenteric adenitis
  Age: older children, adults
  Symptoms: mild diarrhea
               increasing abdominal pain
               signs and symptoms of appendicitis
  Duration: 1–2 wk

(continued)

TABLE 8-36. (continued)

Enterocolitis
   Age: adolescent, young adults
   Symptoms: watery diarrhea
              fever in 50%
   Duration: 2–3 weeks
Collagen—vascular-like disease
   Age: adults
   Symptoms: arthritis
              carditis
              Reiter's syndrome
              erythema nodosum
   Duration: wk to mo
Septicemia
   Age: older adults or immunocompromised (any age)
   Symptoms: spiking fevers
              headache
              vomiting and diarrhea
              malaise, toxic appearing
              metastatic infection
   Duration: as related to involved organs

Yersinia is easily isolated from uncontaminated sources such as joint fluid or blood. It is difficult to isolate on routine stool cultures because it appears as a very small colony which is easily overgrown. Selective media have been developed to allow easy identification of the organism.

Acute gastroenteritis is usually a self-limited disease that does not require therapy. Patients with chronic gastrointestinal symptoms have responded to antibiotics but controlled studies have not been performed. Metastatic infections, such as osteomyelitis or hepatic abscesses, should be treated with antibiotics and the duration of treatment dictated by the site of involvement. Mesenteric adenitis may improve with antibiotic therapy but this is yet unproven. Septicemia is an absolute indication for therapy. Most infections in the United States due to sereotype 0:8 are sensitive to ampicillin and TMP-SMX. European and Canadian strains are sensitive to tetracycline and TMP-SMX. The European strains are generally resistant to most cephalosporins and penicillins due to the production of two distinct β-lactamases. Septicemia is generally treated with aminoglycyosides, chloramphenicol, or TMP-SMX. The duration of therapy in septicemia has not been established; however, several weeks of therapy may be needed (see Chap. 18 for dosages of antibiotics).

Bone and Joint Infections

Infectious agents are introduced into bone by: (a) hematogenous infection from bacteremia, (b) local spread from contiguous foci such as cellulitis or infected varicella lesions, and (c) direct inoculation following trauma, invasive procedures, or surgery. The incidence of osteomyelitis is greater in males (2.5 times more often than females) and approximately 40% of cases occur in patients less than 20 years of age.

HEMATOGENOUS OSTEOMYELITIS

The pathogenesis of hematogenous osteomyelitis begins in the metaphysis of tubular long bones adjacent to the epiphyseal growth plate. Thrombosis of the low velocity sinusoidal vessels due to trauma or embolization is considered the focus for bacterial seeding in this process. This avascular environment allows invading organisms to proliferate while avoiding the influx of phagocytes, the presence of serum antibody and complement, the interaction with tissue macrophages, and other host defense mechanisms. The proliferation of organisms, release of organism enzymes and by-products, and the fixed volume environment contribute to progressive bone necrosis. The signs, symptoms, and pathologic progression is different for newborns, older infants and young children (2 weeks to 4 years of age), and older children and adolescents (4 to 16 years of age).

TABLE 9-1. HEMATOGENOUS OSTEOMYELITIS: SIGNS AND SYMPTOMS

	Newborn	Older Infant and Young Child (2 wk-4 yr)	Older Child and Adolescent (4-16 yr)
Systemic symptoms[a]	Clinical sepsis, irritable, especially to touch; pseudo-paralysis	Pain, limp, refusal to use affected limb	Focal symptoms, less restriction of movement; local pain; mild limp; fever, malaise
Signs	Red, swollen, discolored local site; massive swelling	Marked focality; point tenderness; well localized pain	Focal signs; point tenderness, very localized
Pathology	Thin cortex; dissects into surrounding tissue	Cortex thicker; periosteum dense	Metaphysical cortex thick; periosteum fibrous and dense
Progression	Nidus (purulent) rapidly progresses;[b] subperiosteal	Subperiosteal abscess and edema; metaphyseal involvement	Cortical rupture rare

TABLE 9-1. (continued)

	Newborn	Older Infant and Young Child (2 wk–4 yr)	Older Child and Adolescent (4–16 yr)
Roentgeno- graph	purulence spreads; secondary septic arthritis Useful early— periosteal and bony changes	Later findings confirmatory; early changes—deep soft tissue swelling	Bony changes apparent only after 7–10 days of involvement

[a] May be subclinical; constitutional symptoms (fever, malaise, anorexia, irritability) are no different among the different age groups; also no correlation with severity of constitutional symptoms and ultimate severity of subsequent osteomyelitis.

[b] Residual effects may be anticipated in up to 25% of newborns.

Tubular long bones are primarily involved, especially of the lower extremities; the common sites of bone involvement in children demonstrate this predilection.

TABLE 9-2. SITE OF BONE INVOLVEMENT

Site	Percentage
Femur	36
Tibia	33
Humerus	10
Fibula	7
Radius	3
Calcaneus	3
Ilium	2

The bacterial etiology of hematogenous osteomyelitis demonstrates an age-specific pattern.

TABLE 9-3. BACTERIAL ETIOLOGY IN HEMATOGENOUS OSTEOMYELITIS

Neonate	Infants and Children
Organisms	
Staphylococcus aureus	*S. aureus*
Group B streptococci	Group A streptococci
Escherichia coli	*Haemophilus influenzae*
Proteus sp.	*Salmonella* sp.
Klebsiella sp.	*E. coli*
Salmonella sp.	*P. aeruginosa*
Neisseria gonorrhoeae	*Klebsiella* sp.
Pseudomonas aeruginosa	*Streptococcus pneumoniae*
Candida sp.	*Candida* sp.
	Anaerobes

The differential diagnosis of hematogenous osteomyelitis includes: septicemia, cellulitis, toxic synovitis, septic arthritis, thrombophlebitis, or, in a sickle cell disease patient, a bone infarction. The diagnosis of osteomyelitis is confirmed with isolation of organisms from bone, subperiosteal exudate, or contiguous joint fluid. Needle aspiration through normal skin over involved bone at a subperiosteal site or at the metaphyseal area combined with a potentially involved joint aspiration should be performed by an orthopedic surgeon. Aspirates of involved focal areas yield positive cultures in up to 80 to 85% of cases; the yield of positive blood cultures may be above 50% and should be done routinely prior to initiation of antimicrobial therapy.

The adjunct to microbiologic confirmation is radiologic localization of disease. The diagnosis of osteomyelitis on routine roentgenographs can be subtle to obvious depending on the duration of disease.

TABLE 9-4. ROENTGENOGRAPHIC DIAGNOSIS OF HEMATOGENOUS OSTEOMYELITIS

Day	Changes
0–3	Local, deep soft tissue swelling; near metaphyseal region or with localized findings
3–7	Deep soft tissue swelling; obscured translucent fat lines (spread of edema fluid)
10–21	Variable-bone specific; bone destruction, periosteal new bone formation

The earlier diagnosis of bone involvement has been enhanced with the use of short half-life isotopes such as technetium. The increased uptake on technetium bone scans has two major advantages: completion of procedure with results in 1 to 2 hours and earlier diagnosis at the time of signs and symptoms. A technetium bone scan should be pursued when a patient has obvious evidence of focal pathology, fever of undetermined etiology with historic symptoms and/or an elevated sedimentation rate, or suggestive findings on routine roentgenographs. The bone scan can also aid in directing aspirate procedures for diagnosis and culture. In situations where osteomyelitis is suspected on examination and technetium bone scan but no obvious localization is apparent, secondary radionuclide imaging may be performed. An indium scan using tagged autologous leukocytes requires 24 hours of imaging for completion and is useful in vertebral or pelvic osteomyelitis; gallium scanning requires 24 to 48 hours and may be difficult to read (midline scans) due to uptake in the bowel. Gallium scanning has been suggested to be superior to indium for peripheral osteomyelitis.

TABLE 9-5. SPECIFIC ETIOLOGIES OF OSTEOMYELITIS

Clinical Circumstance	Probable Etiology
Human bite	Anaerobes
Dog or cat bite	*Pasteurella multocida*
Puncture wound of foot	*P. aeruginosa*

(*continued*)

TABLE 9-5. (continued)

Clinical Circumstance	Probable Etiology
Sickle cell disease	*Salmonella* sp.
	Shigella sp.
	E. coli
	Serratia sp.
	Arizona sp.
	Other gram-negative organisms
	Anaerobes
Rheumatoid arthritis	*S. aureus* (from joint)
	P. multocida
Diabetes mellitus	Fungi
Newborns	Group B streptococci
	E. coli
	Salmonella sp.

Uncommon Etiologies	
Facial and cervical area; in the jaw; sinus drainage; lytic bone changes with "egg shell" areas of new bone	*Actinomyces* sp.
Age 3 mo–6 yr (uncommon compared to staphylococci)	*H. influenzae*
Vertebral body or long bone abscesses; systemic signs and symptoms	Brucellosis
Regional distribution; systemic findings; vertebral body, skull, long bone involvement	Coccidioidomycosis
Skin lesions; pulmonary involvement; skull and vertebral bodies most common, but long bone involvement is reported	Blastomycosis
Very distinct, slowly progressive bony lesions can occur	Cryptococcosis

NONHEMATOGENOUS OSTEOMYELITIS

Bone involvement arises through spread from a contiguous focus of infection or direct inoculation. The following are the more common types of nonhematogenous osteomyelitis.

Pseudomonas Osteochondritis

The predilection of *Pseudomonas* to involve cartilaginous tissue and the relative amount of cartilage in children's tarsal-metatarsal region are the reasons for this infection being classified as an "osteochondritis." This entity is seen as early as 2 days postinjury but frequently requires up to 21 days to manifest clinically. The proper initial management of this trauma is vigorous irrigation and cleansing of the puncture wound in conjunction with tetanus prophylaxis. This is frequently overlooked in lieu of simple washing and oral antibiotics ineffective against *Pseudomonas*. Upon diagnosis of *Pseudomonas* osteochondritis from wound, drainage culture or surgical curettage culture, intravenous antibiotics (see Table 9-7) should be initiated and guided by antibiotic sensitivity testing. The crucial factor in successful therapy is complete evacuation of all necrotic, infected bone and cartilage. If this is accomplished, only 7 to 10 days of parenteral antibiotics are necessary (depending on soft tissue healing and appearance) for completion of therapy. *Pseudomonas* osteochondritis of the vertebrae or pelvis should lead one to suspect intravenous drug abuse as an etiology.

Patellar Osteochondritis

Patellar osteochondritis is seen in children 5 to 15 years of age when the patella has significant vascular integrity. Direct inoculation via a puncture wound yields symptoms within 1 week to 10 days whereas constitutional symptoms are uncommon. *Staphylococcus aureus* is the most common etiology. Roentgenographs may take 2 to 3 weeks to show sclerosis or destruction.

Contiguous Osteochondritis

Infection is uncommon in children compared to adults. It is commonly associated with nosocomial-infected burns or penetrating wounds. Two to four weeks frequently precede local pain, skin erosion, ulceration, or sinus drainage. Multiple organisms are common and draining sinus cultures correlate well with bone aspirate or biopsy cultures. *S. aureus*, streptococci, anaerobes in abscesses, and nosocomial gram-negative enterics are the etiologic organisms; peripheral leukocyte count or erythrocyte sedimentation rates are usually normal.

PELVIC OSTEOMYELITIS

The frequency of bone involvement (highest to lowest) is: ilium, ischium, pubis, and sacroiliac areas. The tendency for multifocal involvement is higher in the pelvis compared to other sites. The symptoms may be poorly localized with vague onset; hip and buttock pain with a limp are frequently the only findings. Tenderness to palpation in the buttocks, the sciatic notch, or positive sacroiliac joint findings may be invaluable in this diagnosis. The differential diagnosis includes mesenteric lymphadenitis, urinary tract infection, and acute appendicitis; patients with inflammatory bowel disease have an increased risk for the development of pelvic osteomyelitis.

VERTEBRAL OSTEOMYELITIS

The vertebral venous system with a low flow state and bidirectional flow without valves is likely the predisposing factor of vertebral body osteomyelitis. It is common for two adjacent vertebrae to be involved while sparing the intervertebral disc. Spread to the internal venous system (epidural abscess) or the external venous system (paraspinous abscess) are complications of this infection. The symptoms of vertebral osteomyelitis include constant back pain (usually dull), low-grade fever, and pain on exertion; the signs may include paraspinous muscle spasm, tenderness to palpation or percussion of the spinal dorsal processes, and limitation of motion. The symptoms can frequently be present for 3 to 4 months without overt toxicity or signs of sepsis. Roentgenographs show rarefaction in one vertebral edge as early as several days and progress to marked destruction, usually anteriorly, followed by changes in the adjacent vertebrae and new bone formation. Staphylococci are the infecting organisms in 80 to 90% of cases with gram-negative enterics (associated with UTI), *Pseudomonas* sp. (IV drug abusers), and a small percentage of miscellaneous organisms (see Table 9-3). Parenteral antibiotic therapy for presumed staphylococcal involvement should be initiated with the consideration for a needle aspirate or bone biopsy for culture and sensitivity testing. Antibiotic therapy should be continued for up to 8 weeks but no data are available for the optimal duration; the clinical course should be considered for decisions of therapy beyond this limit. Treatment should also include surgical drainage (especially if cord compression is present) and immobilization (bed rest versus casting).

DISCITIS

Noninfectious disc necrosis versus bacteremic seeding of the disc space during the loss of blood supply are difficult to separate clinically. Intervertebral disc infection demonstrates some important characteristics: male sex predominance, peak incidence under 5 years of age, occurrence nearly always in the lumbar area (L4-L5 then L3-L4 most common), peripheral leukocytosis in only one-third of patients, and consistently elevated ESR. The symptoms include backache, progressive limp, irritability and refusal to sit (nonambulatory infants), hip pain, and low-grade fever. The presence of symptoms has been described from 1 to 18 months duration (median 10 to 12 weeks). The apparent signs may include back stiffness, tenderness to spine palpation, and limitation of movement. *S. aureus* is the most frequent organism; needle aspirate and bone biopsy have been reported as culture positive in up to 50% of cases. Less common isolates include pneumococcus and gram-negative organisms. Roentgenographs (lateral view of lumbar spine) may show disc space narrowing by 2 to 4 weeks after onset of symptoms. This is followed by destruction of adjacent vertebral edges; vertebral body compression is rare. Even with the consideration of noninfectious disc necrosis and the unlikely propensity for dissemination of infection, antibiotics should be started with antistaphylococcal coverage (see Table 9-7). Oral antibiotics are frequently used following 3 to 10 days of parenteral therapy depending on the organism and the clinical situation. Prolonged periods (4 to 6 months) of oral antibiotics may be necessary, depending on the clinical course and extent of damage. The prognosis varies, but, in general, young children reconstitute and heal the disc space whereas older children are more likely to have spontaneous spinal fusion.

TABLE 9-6. SPECIAL CONDITIONS

Closed fractures	Osteomyelitis one to several weeks postfracture; after postfracture pain subsides, the pain recurs with progression; local erythema, warmth, and fluctuation; fever common; osteomyelitis applies to this circumstance
Open fractures	Thorough debridement and wound cleansing paramount; one prospective trial demonstrated a significantly lower infection rate in patients receiving prophylactic first generation cephalosporin for open fractures, the consequence of infection can be significant; staphylococci, streptococci, anaerobes, and *Clostridia* sp. or gram-negative enterics depending on the environment related to the trauma should be considered; tetanus prophylaxis vital (see Chap. 3)
Hemodialysis	Increased risk due to multiple procedures with intravascular cannulae; predisposed involvement of ribs, thoracic spine and bony involvement adjacent to indwelling catheters, *S. aureus* and *S. epidermidis* commonly found

TREATMENT

The treatment of hematogenous osteomyelitis should be guided by gram stain and culture–sensitivities of bone or joint aspirates. Empiric therapy on an age- and disease-related basis administered parenterally should always be initiated (see Table 9–7). The initial use of parenteral antibiotics in acute bacterial hematogenous osteomyelitis is indicated because: physiologic and constitutional changes are not ideal for oral antibiotic absorption; there is propensity for dissemination and abscess formation (especially for *S. aureus*); and compliance in the initial stages when organism proliferation needs to be stopped. Although the route of administration of antibiotics remains controversial, oral absorption is adequate for the continuation of therapy (see Septic Arthritis—Treatment in this chapter). Parenteral therapy should be continued for 3 to 10 days; the total duration of parenteral therapy should be based on evidence of a clinical response. The duration of antibiotic therapy (parenteral and oral) should always be 3 weeks and may have to extend to 4 or 5 weeks depending on the sites of infection and clinical response. (*Pseudomonas* osteochondritis following puncture wound of the foot and surgical debridement is an exception.) Surgical drainage or debridement of subperiosteal abscesses or soft tissue abscesses should never be overlooked. Immobilization of an affected extremity should be considered for pain relief and to enhance healing.

TABLE 9-7. TREATMENT

Infection	Antimicrobial Agents	
Osteomyelitis and septic arthritis		
Empiric Therapy		
Neonate	Methicillin +	ceftriaxone (osteomyelitis)
	Ampicillin +	ceftriaxone (septic arthritis)
Infant	Nafcillin + or cefazolin	cefotaxime ceftizoxime ceftriaxone or chloramphenicol
Children		
< 7 yr	Cefazolin + clindamycin or nafcillin	cefotaxime ceftizoxime ceftriaxone or chloramphenicol
> 7 yr	Cefazolin clindamycin or nafcillin	

(continued)

TABLE 9-7. (continued)

Infection	Antimicrobial Agents
Puncture wound to foot	Gentamicin[a] + tobramycin or amikacin ticarcillin + cefazolin [b] clindamycin or nafcillin

Specific Therapy

S. aureus	Cefazolin, clindamycin, nafcillin, vancomycin (methicillin resistant)
Group B streptococci	Penicillin or ampicillin + gentamicin
Group A streptococci	Penicillin or ampicillin
H. influenzae	Ampicillin (sensitive) or cefotaxime, ceftizoxime, ceftriaxone, chloramphenicol, or moxalactam (ampicillin resistant)
S. pneumoniae	Penicillin or ampicillin (all drugs used in ampicillin resistant H. influenzae effective, except moxalactam)
Enterobacteriaceae	Aminoglycoside; if resistant, azlocillin, mezlocillin, piperacillin or third generation cephalosporins, depending on sensitivities
N. gonorrhoeae	Penicillin or ampicillin; if penicillin resistant, cephalosporin (third generation) or spectinomycin
P. aeruginosa	Aminoglycoside + ticarcillin;
Salmonella sp.	Ampicillin + chloramphenicol
C. albicans	Amphotericin B ± 5-flucytosine
Anaerobes	Penicillin, clindamycin, or metronidazole

Continuation Oral Therapy[c]

S. aureus	Cephalexin, dicloxacillin, oxacillin, or nafcillin
Streptococci	Penicillin or ampicillin
H. influenzae	Ampicillin or amoxicillin, trimethoprim/sulfamethoxazole, erythromycin/sulfasoxazole
S. pneumoniae	Penicillin or ampicillin
Enterobacteriaceae	Ampicillin or trimethoprim/sulfamethoxazole

TABLE 9-7. (continued)

Infection	Antimicrobial Agents
N. gonorrheae	Penicillin or ampicillin
P aeruginosa	No optimal choice currently available
Salmonella sp.	Ampicillin or chloramphenicol
C. albicans	No optimal choice currently available
Anaerobes	Penicillin, metronidazole or clindamycin
Culture negative	Trimethoprim/sulfamethoxazole or Erythromycin/sulfasoxazole

[a] Aminoglycoside choice guided by *Pseudomonas* sensitivities in your hospital.
[b] Concomitant wound infection, Gram stain positive.
[c] Oral continuation (modified by sensitivity testing).

SEPTIC ARTHRITIS

With the production of joint fluid by the synovial membrane, the kinetics of capillary diffusion of fluid into the joint space and the high effective blood flow of the joint space, the relatively high frequency of joint infections is not surprising. Bacteria can enter the joint space by direct inoculation (kneeling on a needle, trauma), contiguous extension (osteomyelitis), or by hematogenous spread. The frequency of joint involvement in children reveals that the lower extremity accounts for at least 80% of cases.

TABLE 9-8. JOINT INVOLVEMENT IN SEPTIC ARTHRITIS

Joint[a]	Percentage
Knee	38
Hip	32
Ankle	11
Elbow	8
Shoulder	5
Wrist	4
Small joints	2

[a] 2–5% of cases have multiple joint involement.

The diagnosis of septic arthritis is made earlier than in osteomyelitis due to the onset of constitutional symptoms within the first few days of the infection. Patients almost always have fever, focal findings in the joint (swelling, tenderness, heat, limitation of motion), and placement of the joint in a neutral, nonstressed position. In infants the hip may have an absence of focal findings with the exception of positioning. Infants are observed with the involved leg abducted, slightly flexed, and externally rotated. Resistance or pain to motion should be evaluated for a possible septic hip. There is often an associated dislocation in this setting. An obvious portal of entry in septic arthritis is rare.

The diagnosis of suspect joint infection by roentgenograms depends on finding evidence of capsular swelling. In the case of hip involvement, roentgenograms can be valuable; placement of the child in the frog-leg position for an anteroposterior radiograph may show displacement of fat lines. Obliteration or lateral displacement of the gluteal fat lines or a raised position for Shenton's line with widening of the arc are consistent with hip joint effusion under pressure. Radionuclide imaging (see Osteomyelitis in this chapter) may be a useful adjunct in a complex or uncharacteristic case for early diagnosis.

The confirmatory procedure for diagnosis is a joint aspiration with gram stain, culture, and cytology-chemistry evaluation. Joint aspiration of knees (most common joint involved) should be a procedure for all primary care physicians; aspiration of hips or shoulders should be limited to an experienced orthopedist (under fluoroscopic control for hip aspirations). Joint fluid should be processed for gram stain and aerobic and anaerobic cultures. The fluid should be analyzed for glucose concentration (compared to a concomitant blood glucose), leukocyte count and differential, ability to spontaneously clot, and mucin clot test. Joint fluid should be obtained in a heparinized syringe to assure leukocyte analysis. To perform the mucin clot test, glacial acetic acid is added to the joint fluid while stirring; normal fluid reacts with a white precipitate (rope) that clings to the stirring rod with a clear supernatant.

TABLE 9-9. JOINT FLUID ANALYSIS

	Septic Arthritis	JRA	Reactive Arthritis
Spontaneous clotting	Large clot	Large clot	Small
Mucin clot	Curdled milk	Small friable masses	Tight rope; clear
Glucose concentration (% of blood glucose)	30	75	75–90
Leukocytes Total	≥ 70,000	15,000	15,000 to 30,000
Leukocytes % PMNs	90	60	∿50

Laboratory diagnosis of septic arthritis can be aided by blood cultures; some series have reported up to 20 to 30% of joint fluids as sterile and blood cultures may yield positive results in these cases. Additional laboratory studies include a hemogram to screen for anemia (hemoglobinopathy), ESR (usually elevated in septic arthritis), serum or urine for bacterial antigen detection (especially in partially treated cases with group B streptococci, *H. influenzae*, pneumococcus, or meningococcus), and accessory cultures. These may include wound cultures, infected skin lesions (secondarily infected varicella lesions over the involved joint), cellulitis aspirate, or urethral-cervical-rectal cultures in sexually active adolescents (gonorrhea). CSF analysis should be included when meningitis is clinically suspected and in all newborns and young infants.

The differential diagnosis of septic arthritis includes joint fluid inflammation due to a variety of etiologies.

TABLE 9-10. DIFFERENTIAL DIAGNOSIS OF SEPTIC ARTHRITIS

Infectious	Viral, mycobacterial, fungal or mycoplasma, bacterial endocarditis, deep cellulitis, Lyme disease, congenital syphilis

(continued)

TABLE 9-10. (continued)

Hypersensitivity	Serum sickness (drug, postinfectious), anaphylactoid purpura
Oncologic	Leukemia, neuroblastoma, pigmented villonodular synovitis, primary bone tumor
Metabolic	Gout, hyperparathyroidism
Immunologic	Agammaglobulinemia, Behçet's syndrome, hepatitis
Neurogenic	Diabetes mellitus, peripheral nerve or spinal cord injury, leprosy
Bleeding	Trauma (to include physical abuse), skeletal trauma due to birth, hemophilia
Orthopedic	Toxic synovitis, aseptic necrosis, osteochondritis, bursitis
Miscellaneous	Kawasaki's syndrome, collagen vascular disease, polyarteritis nodosa, sarcoidosis, inflammatory bowel disease, familial Mediterranean fever, Tietze's syndrome, reactive arthritis

The causative bacteria in most cases of septic arthritis have always been gram-positive aerobic organisms. Although over the past decade *H. influenzae* has been increasing in frequency, *S. aureus* remains the most frequent isolate from infected joints. The causative organisms also differ for neonates, infants, and older children.

TABLE 9-11. ETIOLOGY OF SEPTIC ARTHRITIS

	Newborns and Infants		Young and Older Children
	Community Acquired	*Nosocomial*	*(Combined Series 1941–1975)[a]*
S. aureus	25%	62%	56%
Group B streptococci	52% (50%)	4%	22%

TABLE 9-11. (continued)

	Newborns and Infants		Young and Older Children
	Community Acquired	*Nosocomial*	*(combined series 1941–1975)[a]*
H. influenzae[b]		4%	14%
Pneumococcus			6%
Enterobacteriaceae	5%	13%	7%
Candida sp.		17%	
N. gonorrhoeae	17%		
Miscellaneous[c]	1%	2%	

[a] Multiple series, therefore, total % not 100%.
[b] The most common cause for infants (<2 yr).
[c] Includes *Salmonella* sp. and *Pseudomonas* sp.

TABLE 9-12. SPECIAL CONSIDERATIONS

Neonatal septic arthritis	Subtle presentation
	Unusual organisms
	Use of umbilical catheters
	Difficulty in evaluating hips-shoulders
	Potential catastrophic outcome
Adolescents, monoarticular arthritis	Sexual contact history due to possibility of gonococcal involvement
	Disseminated gonorrhea (perihepatitis, endocarditis, meningitis, sepsis)
Reactive arthritis	Predisposition in HLA-B27 positive patients
	Occurs following *Shigella* sp., *Salmonella* sp., *Yersinia*, and *Campylobacter* enteric infections
	May mimic rheumatic fever, collagen vascular disease, or serum sickness
Reiter's syndrome	Urethritis, conjunctivitis, with or without rash and arthritis (ankles, knees) associated with chlamydia infection

(continued)

TABLE 9-12. (continued)

Lyme disease	Clinical suggestion that early diagnosis and treatment with penicillin may prevent arthritis
Kawasaki syndrome	Arthritis, most common noncardiac complication
	Occurs in 20-30% of cases
	Large joints most common
	Multiple joints
	Respond to salicylates

Treatment

The empiric choice of antimicrobial therapy in septic arthritis should be guided by gram stain or bacterial antigen testing but should consider: *S. aureus* in all cases; increasing incidence of *H. influenzae;* group B streptococci, and to a lesser extent gram-negative organisms and *Candida* sp. in neonates; and *N. gonorrhoeae* in newborns and sexually active adolescents. The other etiologies and age-related incidence include mycoplasma (>10 years), ureaplasma (>5 years), Lyme arthritis (Borrelia-type organism; >6 months), hepatitis B (>1 year), rubella (>10 years), mumps (<12 years), varicella (<5 years) and HSV, CMV, and arboviruses (all ages).

Antibiotic therapy should be directed in cases with negative gram stains-bacterial antigen assays for the most likely organisms that are age-related (see Table 9-7). Nearly all antibiotics that have been studied penetrate readily into joint fluid and average around 30 to 40% of peak serum concentration. The penicillins, cephalosporins (first, second, and third generation), macrolides, aminoglycosides, and chloramphenicol attain effective concentrations in joint fluid. Intraarticular antibiotics add no benefit although irrigation with ingress and egress tubes are effective in joints requiring open drainage. The duration of antibiotic therapy should be 3 weeks minimum with the first 5 to 7 days administered parenterally. The balance of therapy can be administered orally as long as the following criteria are met: no GI disorder or underlying disease that would diminish oral absorption, clinical response to parenteral antibiotics and surgical management has been established; the organism is sensitive to a class of antibiotic in oral form and compliance can be guaranteed. The necessity to administer the oral antibiotics as an inpatient is controversial and should be individualized. For most oral antibiotics, drug level determination can be obtained but is not readily available. The use of a peak serum bactericidal titer and maintenance of this titer at a level of more than or equal to 1:8 is felt to correlate with effective therapy. To evaluate the effectiveness of antibiotic therapy, serial joint aspirations can be performed. Although cultures may be positive for up to 5 to 7 days in nonsurgically drained joint fluid, a decrease in leukocyte density should be seen by 1 to 2 weeks of therapy. In studies using serial joint aspirations, by days 1 through 10 of antibiotic therapy those patients who subsequently recover had less than or equal to 5000 cells/mm^3 compared to those with recrudescent infection who had more than or equal to 60,000 cells/mm^3. The best predictor of outcome and complications is the duration of signs and symptoms prior to diagnosis and effective therapy.

Septic arthritis in neonates and infants, hip or shoulder involvement, is a surgical emergency and should be drained as soon as the diagnosis is established. Any joint should be considered for open drainage when loculation, high fibrin content, or tissue debris prevents adequate drainage by needle aspiration.

Urinary Tract Infections

Urinary tract infections (UTIs) are caused by bacteria that the clinician may identify and treat effectively if a conscientious systematic approach is used. By 10 years of age, the cumulative incidence of UTI is 5% in girls and 1% in boys. Most infections of the urinary tract are ascending in origin. Bacteria from the bowel flora traverse the perineum and the urethra and ultimately colonize the urinary bladder. In males, the greater length of the urethra and the antibacterial properties of prostatic secretions are effective barriers to invasion of the urinary tract. In females a short urethra is the primary reason for their increased frequency of urinary infections.

TABLE 10-1. MECHANISMS OF UTI

Ascending infection
Hematogenous
Lymphogenous
Extension from another organ

Other factors may predispose to the development of UTI. In neonates the source of infection is usually hematogenous and is often associated with urinary tract anomalies. Extension from abdominal infection, such as appendicitis, may occur and lymphatic spread with constipation has been suggested.

TABLE 10-2. FACTORS PREDISPOSING TO UTI

Residual urine
Obstructed urine flow
Vesiculoureteral reflux
Structural abnormalities
Foreign bodies
Nephrolithiasis
Indwelling catheters
Constipation
Poor perineal hygiene

CRITERIA FOR DIAGNOSIS

Symptoms of cystitis may include enuresis, nocturia, or malodorous urine and subside after 24 to 48 hours of effective antibiotic therapy. Fevers are rarely above 38C. Symptomatology, which fails to respond, may be due to less common causes of UTIs.

TABLE 10-3. SYMPTOMS OF LOWER UTI

Urinary	Frequency
	Urgency
	Dysuria
	Daytime dribbling

TABLE 10-3. (continued)

Constitutional	Nocturnal enuresis
	Foul smelling urine
	History of urinary retention
	Fever
	Irritability
	Abdominal pain
	Decreased appetite
Infants	Sepsis
	Lethargy
	Jaundice

The manifestations of UTI are commonly vague and nonspecific; urinary frequency and dysuria are often not reported even by older children. Conversely, half of girls and women presenting with frequency and dysuria do *not* have UTI. Local vaginal or urethral irritation may mimic symptoms of UTI.

TABLE 10-4. CAUSES OF URINARY TRACT SYMPTOMS WITHOUT BACTERIURIA

Urethritis	Vaginal foreign bodies
Vulvovaginitis	Pinworms
Soaps, detergents, bubble bath	*Candida*
Fabrics, laundry soaps, clothing dyes	*Trichomonas*
Medications, lotions	Emotional disturbances
Trauma (sexual abuse)	Frequency-dysuria syndrome (Sham syndrome)

TABLE 10-5. LESS COMMON INFECTIOUS ETIOLOGIES

Virus, e.g., adenovirus
Gonococcus
Chlamydia
Mycoplasma
Anaerobic bacteria

Definitive diagnosis must be based on quantitative cultures of the urine. Criteria for diagnosis of UTI vary according to different methods of collection. A presumptive diagnosis of urinary tract infection may be made on the basis of an abnormal urinalysis, particularly when symptoms and signs of UTI are present. The limitations of presumptive evidence for UTI should be recognized, however.

Pyuria is poorly correlated with infection. Approximately 40% of children with UTI have less than five WBCs per high power field in centrifuged sediment. Conversely, children with pyuria frequently do not have bacteriuria.

TABLE 10-6. CAUSES OF PYURIA WITHOUT BACTERIURIA

Concentrated urine (dehydration)
Irritation from topical agents
Inflammation of neighboring structures, e.g., acute appendicitis
Trauma
Instrumentation
Calculi
Acute glomerulonephritis
Interstitial nephritis
Oral polio vaccine
Renal tubular acidosis

The concentration of leukocytes in a urine sample is increased on centrifuged samples. The volume of urine, the duration and amount of centrifugal force, and the volume of the supernatant fluid influence the amount of leukocytes on microscopic examination. Urine for microscopic evaluation is obtained by spinning 10 ml of urine for 5 minutes at 3000 rpm and counting cells under magnification of 40 times. Other points to remember when making the diagnosis of UTI include:

1. Proteinuria is usually absent in UTI, and children with proteinuria rarely have UTI.

2. Presence of bacteria on a freshly spun urine does correlate with significant bacteriuria.
3. Screening techniques available correlate poorly with the presence of urinary tract infections. Current tests include:
   a. Catalase—an inflammatory enzyme.
   b. Nitrite—bacteria degrade nitrate to nitrite in urine.
   c. Dip slides for culture.

TABLE 10-7. CRITERIA FOR DEFINITIVE DIAGNOSIS OF UTI

Method of Collection	Indeterminant[a]	Positive (Colonies/ml of Urine)
Suprapubic aspiration	Any growth	>100 gram-negative bacilli Gram-positive cocci: >1000
Catheterized urine	10-50,000	>50,000
Clean-voided (male)	≥ 10,000 (fore-skin retracted or absent and glans penis well cleansed)	>100,000
Clean-voided (female)	>50,000	>100,000
Bagged urine	>100,000	

[a] Repeat culture or obtain catheterized or suprapubic sample for culture.

The diagnosis of UTI is only as valid as the care given to the collection of urine for culture. Meticulous attention must be paid to cleaning the perineum, to avoiding vaginal reflux of urine, and to rapid processing of urine samples. Because urine is an excellent culture media for bacteria, all samples must be cultured immediately or refrigerated. Storage of the urine in the refrigerator for as long as 1 week will not alter the quantitative cultures, but failure to refrigerate the specimen within a half hour of collection may lead to falsely high colony counts.

Significant bacteriuria in a urine specimen collected by voiding or catheterization is characterized by high colony counts of a single species of bacteria. The urine that shows squamous and epithelial cells as well as leukocytes probably represents contamination by vaginal reflux or reflux beneath the foreskin. Such a urine should be recollected before being submitted for culture. Contaminated samples usually show low colony counts and/or mixed flora. Bag-collected urine cultures are unreliable and show a high rate of contamination, particularly in female infants.

TABLE 10–8. PRESUMPTIVE EVIDENCE OF CONTAMINATION OF URINE CULTURE

More than one organism
Low colony count
Presence of *Staphylococcus epidermidis*
Low volume voided specimen
Presence of squamous epithelial cells in urinalysis
Improperly collected specimen

Most confusing culture results may be clarified by obtaining a urine sample by catheterization or suprapubic aspiration. Suprapubic aspiration is a relatively atraumatic procedure that causes transient hematuria or other complications in less than 1% of patients (see Chap. 5). The guidelines for colony counts in Table 10-7 give a 90% or greater probability of significant bacteriuria and documentation of UTI. Only 5% of patients with UTI have colony counts as high as 10,000 to 100,000 colonies per milliliter of urine by suprapubic aspiration.

Falsely low colony counts may be found under several circumstances in the specimens from patients who have significant bacteriuria. There may be total inhibition of bacterial growth if a systemic or locally administered bacteriostatic agent is present. Specimens obtained after the child is encouraged to drink liquids to produce a urine specimen are obtained following minimal bladder incubation time and dilution of the urine. A low colony

count may be present in this urine even in the presence of true
bacteriuria.

**TABLE 10-9. CAUSES OF FALSELY LOW COLONY
COUNTS IN PATIENTS WITH
SIGNIFICANT BACTERIURIA**

pH <5.0
Dilute urine (specific gravity < 1.003)
Systemic or topical antimicrobial agents in the urine
Obstruction of urine flow
Pyelonephritis
Fastidious bacteria or *Candida*

Quantitative urine cultures may be obtained in the office using
quantitative bacteriologic loops that deliver approximately 0.001
ml of urine. The methodology is simple and inexpensive. All that
is needed include an alcohol lamp, a quantitative bacteriologic
loop, blood agar plates, and an incubation chamber. The loop is
dipped into urine from a properly collected specimen. Urines,
0.001 ml, are streaked on blood agar plates and incubated from 18
to 24 hours at 37C. Multiplying the number of colonies of bacteria on the blood agar plate by 1000 gives a reasonable approximation of the bacteria per milliliter in the urine specimen. Thus,
more than 100 colonies on a plate is evidence of significant bacteriuria and a quantitative colony count of 10^5 colonies per milliliter.

LOCALIZATION OF UTI

Localization of the site of UTI is difficult and imprecise, yet it is
important to differentiate cystitis (lower UTI) from pyelonephritis (upper UTI). Direct methods of localization are overly invasive. Indirect methods consist of nonspecific measurements of
host response to bacterial infections. The rationale for interpretation of indirect tests is that infections of the renal parenchyma
stimulate the immune system whereas the bladder, an encapsu-

lated externalized organ, does not. Defects in renal concentrating
ability are present in acute and chronic renal parenchymal infections. A normal maximal urinary concentration within a few days
of initiating therapy indicates a lower UTI. Children with pyelonephritis have been found to have higher levels of IgA and IgG
antibodies against Tamm-Horsfal protein, a glycoprotein produced by renal tubular cells, than those with cystitis.

The most reproducible method for localization of UTI in children is measurement of urinary LDH and LDH isoenzymes. Elevation of total urinary LDH and isoenzymes 4 and 5 correlate
with the presence of pyleonephritis. Antibody-coated bacteria
have been used on the assumption that only bacteria that have
invaded the renal parenchyma will be coated by antibodies.
Though the results have been good in adults, in children there is
little correlation between the presence of antibody-coated bacteria and upper UTI. Leukocyte (WBC) casts are a nonspecific
finding that may indicate interstitial nephritis. WBC casts containing bacteria, however, are pathognomonic of bacterial pyelonephritis.

TABLE 10-10. LOCALIZATION OF THE SITE OF URINARY TRACT INFECTION

Direct methods
  Bladder washout
  Ureteral catheterization and culture
  Renal biopsy and culture
Indirect methods
  Nonspecific evidence of infection—CRP, ESR
  Assessment of maximal renal concentrating capacity
  Antibodies to the infecting organism
  Antibodies to Tamm-Horsfal proteins
  Antibody-coated bacteria in urine
  Calculation of leukocyte excretion rates (3-bottle urine collection,
    see Table 10–13)
  Microscopic examination of the urine—WBC casts and bacteria
  Urinary enzyme assays (quantitation of urine LDH isoenzymes)

TABLE 10-11. INTERPRETATION OF TOTAL
URINARY LDH

< 50 suggests lower tract disease
50-150 nondiagnostic; 50:50 chance of upper UTI vs lower UTI
> 150 is highly suggestive of upper UTI
Elevation of fraction 4 and 5 suggestive of upper UTI

TABLE 10-12. CAUSES OF FALSELY ELEVATED
URINARY LDH

Shedding of cells from the kidney
Plasma clearance by glomerular filtration and/or impaired tubular
  resorption
PMN or bacteria in the urine
Secretions of the genital glands
Altered permeability of renal epithelial cell membranes

TABLE 10-13. METHODOLOGY FOR THREE BOTTLE
URINE COLLECTION

Patient voids 5–10 ml into first bottle (urethral washing)
The bladder is emptied into the second bottle (bladder washing)
The patient strains to empty the last 5–10 ml into third bottle
  (prostatic washing)
Samples are sent for quantitative cultures and WBC counts
Interpretation
Increased WBC and colony count in first bottle indicate urethritis
Increased WBC and colony count in second bottle indicate cystitis
Increased WBC and colony count in third bottle indicate prostatitis

BACTERIAL ETIOLOGY

Most UTIs are caused by gram-negative enteric organisms, a
consequence of the ascending of infection from the perineum,
through the urethra to the bladder. Recurrent infections are also
most commonly caused by *Escherichia coli* (70 to 85%), although

other coliforms and *Staphylococcus aureus* are cultured more frequently than from children with initial infections.

TABLE 10-14. ETIOLOGY OF UTI

Organism	Percentage
E. coli	80
Klebsiella-aerobacter	10
Proteus	3
Pseudomonas	1
Enterococcus	1
S. aureus	1

TREATMENT

Antibiotics commonly used to treat lower UTIs are outlined in Table 10-15. Sulfonamide antibiotics should be avoided in neonates with UTI because of competition with bilirubin for albumin binding sites. Most antibiotics are concentrated in the urine to levels 10 to 100 times greater than serum concentrations. This concentration factor greatly enhances and broadens the antibacterial spectrum of most antibiotics and also permits the use of compounds that do not achieve systemic therapeutic concentrations when lower tract disease is being treated.

Antibiotic concentrations used in determining sensitivity by the disc method are chosen on the basis of usual serum concentrations. Thus, in vitro antibiotic resistance may be reported in spite of apparent in vivo elimination of the organism. Sensitivities based on achievable urine concentrations clarify this misinterpretation.

Bacteriuria is usually eradicated in 24 to 48 hours after initiation of effective antimicrobial therapy. Pyuria may persist longer. Thus, a shorter duration of treatment than the standard 10 to 14 days may be effective in most cases of lower UTIs. Because most pharmacies have a minimum prescription charge, single dosage or short-term antibiotic therapy may not be cost effective.

Warm sitz baths for 20 to 30 minutes, three to four times a day, usually relieve symptoms of urgency, frequency, and mild urinary retention. Topical analgesics, such as phenazopyridine, which may stain underclothes or temporarily stain the oral mucosa in patients who chew the tablets, are usually not needed.

TABLE 10-15. ANTIBIOTICS RECOMMENDED FOR TREATMENT OF ACUTE LOWER UTI

Antibiotics	Dosage
Amoxicillin	20-30 mg/kg/day, div q8h
Ampicillin	50-100 mg/kg/day, div q6h (maximum 2 g/day)
Sulfisoxazole	120-150 mg/kg/day div q6h (maximum 2 g/day)
Nalidixic acid	55 mg/kg/day, div q6h (maximum 4 g/day)
Nitrofurantoin	5-7 mg/kg/day, div q6h (maximum 400 mg/day)
TMP-SMX	6-12 mg of trimethoprim, 30-60 mg of SMX/kg/day, div q12h
Cephalexin	25-50 mg/kg/day, div q6h (maximum 2 g/day)

TABLE 10-16. UNIQUE ASPECTS OF ANTIBIOTICS FOR UTI

Antibiotics	Comment
Nitrofurantoin	Acid urine essential (pH<5.5)
	Not recommended in neonates or uremia
	Available in IV form
	Bowel flora resistance develops slowly
	Nausea and vomiting common in infants; can cause hemolytic anemia
Methenamine	Acid urine essential (pH<5.5)
	Hydrolyzed to formaldehyde
	Supplement with ascorbic acid (1 g/day)
	Limit urine output to 1000 ml/day
Nalidixic acid	Resistance develops rapidly
	Gives false positive urine dipstick for glucose

TABLE 10–17. ANTIBIOTICS FOR TREATMENT OF
ACUTE PYELONEPHRITIS

Antibiotic	Daily Dosage[a]
Gentamicin	7.5 mg/kg div q8h
Ampicillin	100 mg/kg div q6h
Tobramycin	5 mg/kg div q8h
Carbenicillin	400 mg/kg div q6h
Ticarcillin	300 mg/kg div q6h
Piperacillin	200 mg/kg div q6h

[a] See Chapter 18 for dosage in neonates.

RECURRENT UTI

Recurrent infections are observed in 30 to 50% of children with UTI with approximately 90% of these occurring within 3 months of the initial episode. Eighty percent of recurrences are new infections by different fecal-colonic bacterial species that have become resistant to recently administered antibiotics. The recurrence rate is not altered by extending the duration of treatment.

The anatomic status of the upper urinary tract or the presence or absence of vesiculoureteral reflux can have an important bearing on the long-term treatment chosen in recurrent UTI. Children who have more than two UTIs in a 12-month period may need chronic suppressive antibiotic therapy for 3 to 6 months to allow repair of intrinsic bladder defense mechanisms. Girls with frequent UTIs tend to have asymptomatic recurrences. Children with recurrent UTI and anatomic defects or reflux may need suppressive antibiotics for as long as the defect exists. Resistance to antibiotics commonly develops, however, due to R_1 factors in fecal-colonic bacteria in patients on long-term suppressive therapy.

Other methods for decreasing reinfections of the lower urinary tract include avoiding bubble bath and detergents in the bath water, wiping the perineal area from front to back after voiding

or defecation, ingesting 1 to 2 quarts of water each day, emptying
the bladder every 3 to 4 hours during the day, and wearing cotton
panties that have no permanent or aniline dyes.

TABLE 10-18. PREVENTION OF RECURRENT UTI

Antibiotics	Daily Dosage
TMP-SMX	2 mg of TMP/10 mg of SMX/kg as a single bedtime dose
Sulfisoxazole	10-20 mg/kg div q12h
Methenamine mandelate	75 mg/kg div q6h
Nitrofurantoin	1-2 mg/kg div q12h

PERSISTENT UTI
Failure to eradicate an organism from the urine suggests an anatomic or physiologic defect. These patients require suppressive
antibiotics until the underlying abnormality resolves (usually 4 to
6 weeks) or is corrected surgically.

TABLE 10-19. FACTORS CAUSING PERSISTENT UTI

Residual urine—neurogenic bladder or anatomic defects
Foreign bodies—catheters, stones
Vesiculoureteral reflux
Static urine flow

INDICATIONS FOR RADIOLOGIC EVALUATION
Radiologic evaluation of the urinary tract should be undertaken
after the first infection in all females less than 3 years of age and
in any patient with evidence of pyelonephritis. All males, regardless of age should be evaluated on their first UTI. Over 3 years of
age females should be evaluated after their second UTI. Initial

evaluation should include an intravenous pyelogram or ultrasound of the kidneys and a VCUG. Ideally the VCUG should be
performed 6 weeks after the acute infection. There is no indication for cystoscopy or urethral dilation. In anatomically normal
kidneys, repeat intravenous pyelograms are only indicated after 3
to 5 years. VCUG should be repeated annually if there is evidence of abnormal bladder anatomy, abnormal bladder function,
or vesiculoureteral reflux.

**TABLE 10–20. INDICATIONS FOR INITIAL
RADIOGRAPHIC STUDIES**

Females
   Initial infection
     <3 yr of age
     pyelonephritis at any age
   Second infection
     >3 yr of age
     not indicated for sexually active females unless pyelonephritis
       is documented
Males
   With initial infection at all ages

VESICULOURETERAL REFLUX

The important anatomic features of the normal vesiculoureteral
valve mechanism include the oblique entry of the ureter into the
bladder wall and the length of the submucosal segment of the intramural ureter. The passive compression of the intramural ureter
by increased intravesicular pressure prior to and during mictura-
tion and the contraction of the ureteral trigonal longitudinal
muscles close the ureteral meatus and the submucosal tunnel.
With vesiculoureteral reflux the submucosal segment is short or
absent and the longitudinal muscles around the submucosal ureter are deficient. Therefore, during voiding, pressure from the
bladder can force urine through an incompetent valve and up-
ward toward the kidney. Vesiculoureteral reflux of infected urine

from the bladder into the renal pelvis is the primary cause of pyelonephritis in children.

The natural course of vesiculoureteral reflux in children is improvement with age. Vesiculoureteral reflux is graded radiographically according to the distance contrast media travels. Over 75% of grades I and II reflux resolve with prophylactic antibiotic therapy. Grade III reflux is observed more often because (5 to 15%) in neonates and infants less pressure is required to produce intrarenal reflux in young children. Grades III and IV reflux may be associated with significant renal damage. Only 25% of Grade III reflux spontaneously resolves without ureteral tailoring and/or surgical reimplantation. Children with vesiculoureteral reflux should receive annual VCUGs until the reflux resolves. In the abscence of significant anatomic abnormalities, repeating the intravenous pyelogram after 4 to 5 years is usually adequate. If the child with vesiculoureteral reflux and UTI has no renal scarring by age 5 years it is unlikely that scarring will occur later, even though the reflux persists. The younger child, those with recurrent pyelonephritis, and those with poorly controlled infections are more likely to develop renal parenchymal damage. Biannual and annual VCUGs or nucleotide cystograms and an intravenous pyelogram every 1 to 2 years may be appropriate in these children. The incidence of significant renal abnormalities or reflux is very low in sexually active adolescents.

FREQUENCY—DYSURIA (SHAM) SYNDROME

Some patients have repeated episodes with symptoms of UTIs but do not have significant bacteria on culture. Noninfective etiologies such as bubble bath or dishwashing detergent in the bath water, instrumentation, local ulcers, diaper rashes, sexual intercourse, or masturbation must be investigated (see Table 10-4). Though an occasional patient has abnormal voiding patterns from a bladder diverticulum or muscle inoordination, "urethral stenosis" as a cause of UTI is extremely rare and urethral dilation or cystoscopy is seldom indicated.

If there is a question of bacteriuria, suprapubic aspiration or bladder catheterization is indicated. If less than 10^5 bacteria are grown from a clean voided specimen, *Chlamydia*, mycoplasma, or local irritation should be suspected. An occasional patient with less than 10^5 staphylococci on culture will respond to appropriate antibiotic therapy. Most cases respond to symptomatic relief with warm sitz baths three to four times daily and analgesic agents such as aspirin, acetaminophen, or phenazopyridine (Pyridium).

CANDIDURIA

UTIs due to *Candida* are uncommon in normal patients. Predisposing conditions to fungal infections include those that alter the normal bacterial suppression of fungal overgrowth, such as antibiotic therapy and decrease in host defense mechanisms, such as debilitation, corticosteroid therapy, or immunosuppression. Mechanical contamination during surgery, especially from Foley catheterization or factors that cause glucosuria, residual urine, or lowered urinary pH also increase the incidence of candiduria (Table 10-21).

Symptoms unique to candiduria include the obstruction of urine flow by fungal balls in cases of candida pyelonephritis. Diagnosis is confirmed by culture of greater than 10,000 colonies per milliliter of Candida on a clean catch urine or by ultrasonographic demonstration of fungus balls in the renal pelvis.

If infection is localized to the bladder, local irrigation with 100 to 300 ml of a solution of amphotericin B, (5 to 15 mg/100 ml D_5W) can be curative. Fluid is instilled into the bladder; the catheter is clamped for 60 to 120 minutes, and the bladder drained. Irrigation is performed three or four times a day for 2 to 5 days. Removal or changing indwelling Foley catheter is mandatory and often curative without antifungal therapy.

A short course (5 to 10 days) of systemic antifungal agents may be needed for the immune compromised host and given according to recommendations for systemic fungal infection. Amphotericin B, flucytosine, and ketoconazole all reach fungicidal levels in the urine.

TABLE 10–21. CONDITIONS THAT PREDISPOSE TO DEVELOPMENT OF CANDIDA UTI

Indwelling catheters
Debilitation
Diabetes mellitus
Immunosuppression
Corticosteroids
Chronic antibiotic therapy

TABLE 10–22. TREATMENT OF CANDIDURIA

Removal or change catheter
Bladder irrigation with amphotericin B 15 mg/100 ml D_5W
Systemic antifungal agents
    Amphotericin B 0.3 mg/kg/day IV div qd × 2-5 days
    Flucytosine 50-150 mg/kg/day PO div q8h
    Ketoconazole 5 mg/kg/day PO div q12h

PERINEPHRIC ABSCESS

This infection may present as an acute abdomen or have a more insidious onset. Perinephric abscesses are usually secondary to the extension of a renal parenchymal infection and are located between the renal capsule and the perirenal fascia. The causative organisms are usually gram-negative rods. Physical examination reveals CVA tenderness and a bulging mass in the flank. Diagnosis is made by ultrasonography, pyelography, or arteriography. The psoas shadow is usually absent on abdominal films. Treatment is the same as for acute pyelonephritis.

RENAL CARBUNCLE

A renal carbuncle can be distinguished from a perinephric abscess by induration of the skin and the presence of a multilocular abscess. This infection is most commonly a consequence of extension from a cutaneous abscess. The causative organism is usually *S. aureus*. Renal carbuncles may rupture into the perirenal or retroperitoneal space. Symptoms and therapy are similar to perinephric abscess.

Genital Tract Infections

Female
   Vulvovaginitis
   Vaginitis
Male
   Balanitis
   Epididymitis
   Prostatitis
   Orchitis

FEMALE

Vulvovaginitis

Prepubertal vaginitis is usually secondary to *Candida albicans*, *Trichomonas vaginalis*, *Neisseria gonorrhoeae*, foreign bodies, or irritation secondary to chemicals or pinworm; it may, however, be the only physical finding in sexual abuse. Gonococcal vaginitis in the prepubertal child is usually mild because it is localized to the superficial mucosa.

The major symptoms include vaginal itching and a minor crusting discharge that discolors the child's underwear. Dysuria and pyuria are common. The character of the vaginal discharge in all patients and the speculum examination in postpubertal (especially sexually active) females are useful in establishing the diagnosis. The treatment of vulvovaginitis in prepubertal and postpubertal females is dependent on the etiologic agent.

TABLE 11-1. VULVOVAGINITIS: CLINICAL CONSIDERATIONS

Clinical Examination	Vaginal Discharge

Ectropion
  PO contraceptives
  Pregnancy
	Clear mucus

Cervicitis (GC, *Chlamydia,* HSV)	Purulent exudate, cervix friable
Vaginitis (*Candida, Trichomonas, Gardnerella vaginalis*)	Malodor, yellow to white, frothy, cervicitis may be present

Vaginitis

A thorough speculum examination is important to ascertain whether the discharge emanates from the vagina or the cervical os. The most common etiologies of vaginitis are: candida, trichomonas, and *Gardnerella vaginalis.* In candida vaginitis the following are helpful in diagnosis: itching, dysuria, curds or plaques, 10% KOH-no odor, yeast, or pseudomycelia, pH of less than 4.5, and a culture positive for yeast. In vaginitis due to trichomonas the diagnosis is apparent with profuse, yellow-green discharge, 10% KOH-amine odor, motile trichomonads (wet preparation, 400×), and a vaginal pH of 5.5 to 6.0. In nonspecific vaginitis, *G. vaginalis,* the diagnosis is apparent with an adherent homogenous discharge, thin, 10% KOH-amine odor, clue cells (secretions in a 1:1 dilution in normal saline), which are vaginal epithelial cells coated with coccobacillary forms of *G. vaginalis,* a pH of more than 4.5, and a positive culture. In some cases of vaginitis, anaerobes have been isolated but no predominant organism has been demonstrated. For comparison, normal vaginal secretions have no odor with 10% KOH and a pH of less than 4.5.

TABLE 11-2. VULVOVAGINITIS—TREATMENT

Candida	Discontinue antibiotics and oral contraceptives if possible. Topical antifungals: nystatin vaginal tablet bid

TABLE 11-2. (continued)

	× 7 days, or imidazole (clotrimazole or miconazole): intravaginally qd × 7 days
Trichomonas	Metronidazole 10-30 mg/kg/day maximum 2.0 g PO single dose or 250 mg PO tid × 10 days
	Alternative—Tinidazole 2.0 g PO single dose
	In pregnancy—Clotrimazole 2-100 mg vaginal tablets at bedtime × 7 days
	Neonatal trichomoniasis—Symptomatic or persistent colonization, metronidazole 10-30 mg/ kg/day PO for 5-8 days
Nonspecific vaginitis (*G. vaginalis*)	Metronidazole 10-30 mg/kg/day maximum 500 mg PO bid × 7 days
	Alternative—ampicillin 50 mg/kg/day maximum 500 mg PO qid × 7 days (pregnancy)
	Sexual partners—Controversial, recommend treatment as in the female

MALE

Balanitis

The characteristic erosive soreness and ulceration of the glans penis develops 6 to 24 hours after sexual intercourse in which the partner invariably has vaginal candidiasis. There are two types of candidal balanitis considered to be of clinical significance.

TABLE 11-3. CANDIDAL BALANITIS

Type	Characteristics	Treatment
Invasive	Soreness, ulceration of the glans penis, marked phimosis,	Nystantin ointment 100,000 U/g, applied qid until *(continued)*

TABLE 11-3. (continued)

Type	Characteristics	Treatment
Hypersensitivity	discharge from under the prepuce	resolved; treat sexual partner
	Primary irritant effect secondary to contact	Good hygiene; treat sexual partner

Balanitis secondary to *Trichomonas* or *G. vaginalis* presents as a nondescript episode of irritation, soreness, pruritic rash, or crusting with occasional dysuria. The best method for diagnosis is direct examination of the first aliquot of a voided urine and if negative, examination of female sexual contact. Treatment for symptomatic males and asymptomatic contacts are identical.

TABLE 11-4. BALANITIS—TREATMENT

Type	Treatment
Trichomonas	Children—Metronidazole 10-30 mg/kg/day PO tid × 7 days
	Adult—Metronidazole 2.0 g PO single dose or 250 mg tid × 7 days
G. vaginalis	Children—Metronidazole 10-30 mg/kg/day PO tid × 7 days
	Adult—Metronidazole 500 g PO bid × 7 days
	Alternative—Ampicillin 500 mg PO qid × 7 days

Other unusual causes of balanitis are related to postcircumcision wound infections. Pathology is similar to cellulitis, impetigo, or burns and should be treated accordingly.

Epididymitis

Epididymitis must be differentiated from testicular torsion, orchitis, or testicular cancer. Acute epididymitis in adolescents usually occurs after trauma and/or heavy lifting and is rarely a primary infection. Epididymitis is suspected when scrotal edema is associated with the presence of fever; pain is relieved by elevation of the scrotum. Ultrasonography in acute epididymitis shows the swollen epididymis represented by distinct parallel lines posterolateral to the discrete testicular echo and an enlarged but separate epididymal head. In torsion of the testis, the testicular echo is disrupted and the echogenic epididymis is inseparable from the testis. Because differentiating acute epididymitis from torsion of the testicle is difficult in teenage boys, surgical exploration is usually indicated. Urine culture may isolate the causative organism. Mumps orchitis is suspected by the lack of WBC in the urine of these patients, a negative culture, and an elevated serum amylase.

Scrotal elevation by an athletic supporter or towel across the thighs facilitates drainage and relief of pain. Sexual excitement may exacerbate pain and infection. Antibiotics are helpful but not curative. Severe pain may be relieved by infiltrating the spermatic cord in the upper scrotum with 1 to 2 ml of 1% xylocaine. Prolonged infection may lead to abscess formation. In cases with prolonged induration of the scrotum, percutaneous biopsy should be avoided. Rather, exploration and open biopsy are indicated to distinguish testicular tumors and to avoid spread of malignant cells.

TABLE 11-5. CAUSES OF ACUTE EPIDIDYMITIS

Preexisting prostatitis
Traumatic reflux of urine
Postprostatectomy

Prostatitis
Acute prostatitis is associated with a purulent urethral discharge and symptoms of dysuria, frequency, and urgency. There may be perineal aching or low back pain. Symptoms are usually more pronounced at the initiation or termination of voiding. Rectal ex-

amination reveals an exquisitely tender, firm prostate. Prostatic massage is not indicated in acute prostatitis. A three-bottle urine collection shows increased WBC in the third voided specimen (see Table 10-13). There is some evidence that two antibiotics, erythromycin, and trimethoprim, are more active in prostate tissue. Most infections are treated with antibiotics commonly used for UTIs. However, symptomatic relief may be obtained by analgesics and warm sitz baths.

TABLE 11-6. ANTIBIOTIC THERAPY FOR ACUTE PROSTATITIS

Antibiotics	Dosage
Tetracycline	2 g/day div q6h × 14 days
Ampicillin	2 g/day div q6h × 14 days
TMP–SMX	160 mg TMP/800 mg SMX/day div q12h × 14 days (treat 3 mo for chronic infection)
Erythromycin	2 g/day div q6h × 14 days

Orchitis

Mumps orchitis is usually associated with parotitis. Although the virus is excreted in the urine, urinalysis is normal. Serum amylase is elevated in these patients.

One third to one fourth of patients with mumps orchitis develop oligo or aspermatism in the involved testis. The other testis is normal and potency is not affected. Treatment is symptomatic with analgesics and elevation.

Skin and Soft Tissue Infections

Acne
Adenopathy
Blepharitis
Decubitis Ulcers
Exanthematous Diseases
Hordeolum and Chalazion
Impetigo
Lacerations and Puncture Wounds
Ludwig's Angina
Molluscum Contagiosum
Myositis
Scabies
Scrofula
Warts (Verrucae)

Skin and soft tissue infections occurring in the normal child are usually easily managed with debridement and good personal hygiene. When therapy is considered necessary, local care (topical) and/or systemic antibiotics are the treatments most commonly used. Persistent or severe infections should alert the physician to the possibility of other underlying conditions.

ACNE

Acne is a common skin condition of adolescence. The pathogenesis of this skin disease is poorly understood. Two microorganisms thought to be associated with this condition are *Propionibacterium acnes* and *Staphylococcus epidermidis*.

TABLE 12–1. TREATMENT OF ACNE

Systemic	Antibiotics (tetracycline has been the most frequently prescribed but erythromycin is also acceptable)
	Steroids have also been used in severe cases
Topical	Trans-retinoic acid (tretinoin 0.01–0.1%) to remove comedones
	Benzoyl peroxide in combination with trans-retinoic acid
	Clindamycin hydrochloride solution
Diet	No effective dietary therapy has been documented, however, good nutrition should be maintained
Surgery	Manual expression of comedones
	Incision and drainage of infected areas is rarely indicated
	Injection of triamcinolone acetonide into cysts may be helpful

ADENOPATHY

Lymph node involvement in children may reflect either a localized infection or a generalized systemic process. Multiple bacteria have been recognized as etiologic agents of adenitis and therapy should be aimed at these organisms (see Table 4-4). Diagnosis may require needle aspiration or biopsy.

When adenopathy is persistent, there are other important diagnostic considerations, both infectious and noninfectious. Most important is ruling out diagnoses where early intervention is of major clinical benefit.

TABLE 12-2. CAUSES OF PERSISTENT OR GENERALIZED ADENOPATHY

Infectious
   Tuberculosis (scrofula)
   Infectious mononucleosis
   CMV
   Toxoplasmosis
   Other viruses
   Tularemia
   Kawasaki disease
   Syphilis
   Hepatitis
   Brucellosis
Noninfectious
   Leukemia
   Lymphoma
   Neuroblastoma
   Other malignancies
   Sarcoidosis

With persistent adenopathy, the primary concern centers around the possibility that an oncogenic process may be the etiology. If the patient is younger than 8 years of age, leukemia is the most likely malignancy and this can be screened with a simple CBC. If the child is older than 8 years, lymphoma is a possibility and can only be ruled out with an excisional biopsy. Prior to this procedure, other aspects of the differential diagnosis may be evaluated during a 30-day observation period as outlined below.

TABLE 12-3. APPROACH TO PERSISTENT ADENOPATHY

Initial evaluation
   History (pertinent exposure)
   Physical examination (measure lymph nodes; if fluctuant see
     Table 4-4)

(continued)

TABLE 12-3. (continued)

CBC
Mono spot test
TB skin test
Throat culture
Chest x-ray
Serum to hold (acute serum)
Initial management (above laboratory results negative)
  Penicillin V 250 mg PO q6h × 14 days
  Remeasure node in 14 days
14 days
  Node smaller: no further evaluation
  Node unchanged, larger or additional nodes:
    Repeat mono spot test
    Second strength PPD
    Serum (convalescent, paired with acute)
      EBV
      CMV
      toxoplasma
30 days (all tests negative)
  Excisional biopsy

BLEPHARITIS

Recurrent inflammation of the eyelid margins frequently occurs in persons with poor personal hygiene or hypersensitivity. Complaints include redness, irritation, and burning. Diagnosis may require culture and scrapings from the inflamed eyelid margins. Gram stains demonstrate PMN leukocytes and bacteria.

TABLE 12-4. ETIOLOGIC AGENTS OF BLEPHARITIS

S. aureus
Moraxella lacunata
Pediculus pubis
Pediculus capitis
Demodex follicularum

Treatment consists of daily debridement with warm, moist compresses and generalized improved personal hygiene. Topical antibiotic ophthalmic drops (sulfacetamide, bacitracin, chloramphenicol, or gentamicin) may be used three to four times per day. Local corticosteriods are employed for allergic blepharitis. Systemic antibiotics are only necessary in resistant cases.

For pediculus infestation, remove the parasites and ova with forceps and apply 3% ammoniated mercury ointment or 1% physostigmine ointment four times per day for 7 days. Another alternative is petrolatum, two or three times daily for 7 to 8 days. Other areas of infestation must also be treated.

DECUBITUS ULCERS

Decubitus ulcers occur when soft tissues have suffered prolonged pressure, friction, and shearing force. Pressure over body sites first results in erythema. Once skin and soft tissue breakdown progresses, bacterial colonization and subsequently deeper invasion occur. Bacterial etiology can be determined by standard culture techniques. Occasionally biopsy is required to obtain meaningful culture material.

TABLE 12-5. MOST COMMON SITES OF DECUBITUS ULCERS

Sacrum
Heel
Ischium
Lateral malleolus

TABLE 12-6. ETIOLOGIC AGENTS RECOVERED FROM DECUBITUS ULCERS

S. aureus
S. epidermidis
Gram-negative enterics
Anaerobic organisms

TABLE 12-7. TREATMENT OF DECUBITUS ULCERS

Relieve pressure, friction, and shearing force
Removal of devitalized tissues
Keep surrounding areas of skin clean and dry
Topical and systemic antibiotics should be selected on the basis of
culture and sensitivity patterns and used only for more severe
cases

EXANTHEMATOUS DISEASES
The exanthematous diseases may be difficult to diagnose. Features to consider include: immunization history, exposure, prodromal period, nature and distribution of rash, diagnostic and pathognomonic signs, and laboratory confirmation.

TABLE 12-8. CLASSIFICATION OF RASHES

Maculopapular
  Miliaria
  Measles
  Rubella
  Scarlet fever
  Enteroviral
  Infectious mononucleosis
  Erythema infectiosum
  Exanthem subitum
  Toxoplasmosis
Kawasaki disease
Scalded-skin (staphylococcus)
Meningococcemia
Rocky Mountain spotted fever
  other tick fevers
Typhus
Toxic erythemas
Drug eruption
Sunburn
Papulovesicular
  VZV
  Coxsackie virus infections
  Rickettsialpox

Papulovesicular (*cont.*)
  Disseminated herpes simplex
  Impetigo
  Insect bites
Petechial
  Rocky Mountain spotted
   fever
  Meningococcemia
  Measles (atypical)
  Infectious mononucleosis
  Haemophilus influenzae sepsis
Papular urticaria
  Drug eruptions
  Molluscum contagiosum

HORDEOLUM AND CHALAZION

A hordeolum is an infection of the glands of Zeis. Most frequently it results from a staphylococcal infection of the ciliary follicle and associated sebaceous glands.

A chalazion is a granulomatous process caused by retention of Meibomian gland secretions. Although it usually resolves spontaneously, excision is occasionally required.

TABLE 12-9. TREATMENT OF HORDEOLUM AND CHALAZION

Hordeolum	Warm compresses
	Topical antistaphylococcal ointment
	Resistant cases may require incision and drainage and systemic antibiotics
Chalazion	Similar to hordeolum but may require excision

IMPETIGO

Impetigo is a superficial infection of the skin caused by group A streptococcus. *S. aureus* as a secondary agent is frequently recovered with streptococcus. The localized skin infection may follow minor trauma. The disease first appears as a discrete papulovesicular lesion surrounded by erythema. Lesions become purulent and form an amber-colored crust. These lesions are contagious and care must be taken to prevent spread to other individuals.

TABLE 12-10. TREATMENT OF IMPETIGO

Careful cleansing with soap and water
Penicillin V PO <60 lbs 125 mg q6h × 10 days
              >60 lbs 250 mg q6h × 10 days
In penicillin-sensitive patients: erythromycin 35-50 mg/kg/day div q6h (maximum 1 g/day) × 10 days

LACERATIONS AND PUNCTURE WOUNDS

Trauma to the skin and soft tissues, either by way of laceration or puncture wound, has the potential to develop secondary bacterial infection. Often the most likely bacterial etiology depends on the nature of the wound and location (i.e., *Staphylococcus* and *Streptococcus* with lacerations and *Pseudomonas* with puncture wounds to the feet). Therefore, appropriate antibiotic therapy depends on assessment as to the most likely organism and the development of secondary infection.

TABLE 12-11. TREATMENT OF LACERATIONS AND PUNCTURE WOUNDS

Irrigation
Careful debridement and removal of foreign material
Suturing as indicated to prevent fluid collection
Antibiotics should be used only if infection has occurred
Initiate tetanus prophylaxis as indicated

LUDWIG'S ANGINA

Lugwig's angina is an extensive, rapidly progressing cellulitis of the floor of the mouth. Although rarely seen today, it can be a serious infection leading to sepsis and/or airway obstruction, and requires immediate medical intervention. Diagnosis by needle aspiration is recommended for bacterial culture.

TABLE 12-12. ETIOLOGIC AGENTS CAUSING LUDWIG'S ANGINA

Staphylococcus
Pneumococcus
H. influenzae
E. coli
Pseudomonas
Neisseria
Fusiform bacilli
Anaerobic streptococcus

TABLE 12–13. TREATMENT OF LUDWIG'S ANGINA

Control the infection and maintain the airway
Intravenous antibiotics (penicillinase-resistant penicillin and
  chloramphenicol or a third generation cephalosporin)
Surgical drainage if fluctuation is present

MOLLUSCUM CONTAGIOSUM

Molluscum contagiosum is a disease of the skin caused by a pox
virus. It appears that the virus is spread by direct contact and
sexual abuse is one consideration in the infected child. Diagnosis
is established by biopsy, stained smears of the expressed molluscum body, or viral cultures.

TABLE 12–14. TREATMENT OF MOLLUSCUM CONTAGIOSUM

Extraction or curettage
Liquid nitrogen freezing
Topical application of cantharidin collodion

MYOSITIS

Myositis is inflammation of large muscle. It may be preceded by
local trauma. Muscle pain is usually the initial symptom, followed by local swelling. Diagnosis may be made by needle aspiration, blood cultures, or muscle biopsy.

TABLE 12–15. ETIOLOGY OF MYOSITIS

Bacteria
  S. aureus
  Group A β-hemolytic streptococci

(continued)

TABLE 12-15. (continued)

Viruses
    Influenza B
    Coxsackie B
    Herpes simplex
Parasites
    Cysticercosis
    Toxoplasmosis
    Trichinosis

TABLE 12-16. TREATMENT OF MYOSITIS

Therapy is determined by etiologic agent (usually systemic
  penicillinase-resistant penicillin: nafcillin)
Incision and drainage
Analgesics as needed

SCABIES

Sarcoptes scabiei, the itch mite, causes a pruritic rash when the skin has been invaded. Classically, the lesions involve the sides and webs of the fingers, flexor surface of the wrist, elbow, anterior axillary folds, female breast, abdomen, penis, and buttocks. In infants and younger children atypical sites, such as the scalp, neck, palms, and soles, may be involved.

Identification of the mite in skin scrapings is accomplished by placing a drop of mineral oil on a suspected lesion and scraping the lesion with a scalpel blade. The scrapings are examined under the light microscope.

Shower and shampoo prior to treatment. Apply to the entire body, sparing the face: 1% gamma benzene hexachloride (Kwell) or, crotamiton (Eurax); rub in gently. It should be left on for 12 hours and then carefully washed off. Repeat treatment is only needed should reinfection occur. Bed linens and clothes need laundering at the start of treatment. All infected family members should be simultaneously treated.

265

SCROFULA

Tuberculosis of lymph nodes and overlying skin is called scrofula. Cervical lymph nodes are most frequently involved. *Mycobacterium tuberculosis* or atypical mycobacteria (*M. kansasii* or *M. marinum*) are commonly identified agents.

Scrofula may resolve spontaneously without therapy. The treatment of choice for persistent nodes is excisional biopsy. Specific chemotherapy depends upon the sensitivity of isolated agents. Often these microorganisms are resistant to standard antituberculous therapy. Rifampin and ethambutol have been used with some success.

WARTS (VERRUCAE)

Warts or verrucae are a common viral disease of the skin caused by a papavavirus. Transmission is thought to be by direct contact.

Spontaneous resolution may occur. Topical application of podophyllin, 40% salicylic acid, 90% trichloroacetic acid, electrodesiccation, or liquid nitrogen freezing are usually curative.

Central Nervous System Infections

BRAIN ABSCESS AND CEREBRITIS

The diagnosis and management of intracranial bacterial suppurative disease has evolved remarkably with the advent of CT and newer antibiotics. Brain abscess, subdural empyema, and other suppurative intracranial disorders, however, remain life-threatening and are frequently associated with significantly disabling neurologic deficits.

Brain abscesses begin as focal bacterial encephalitis or cerebritis characterized by neutrophilic infiltration and edema. Over several days fibroblastic proliferation and increased vascularity surround an increasingly necrotic core of liquified brain tissue, forming the "encapsulated" abscess. Contiguous or hematogenous spread of infection often superimposed over significant host factors contributes to clinically recognizable patterns. Typically brain abscesses from contiguous spread develop adjacent to the initiating site. Those abscesses from hematogenous spread frequently occur in a middle cerebral artery distribution.

TABLE 13-1. FACTORS PREDISPOSING TO BRAIN ABSCESS

Contiguous spread
  Sinusitis
    Frontal
    Ethmoidal
  Mastoiditis and otitis media
  Trauma
    Cribriform plate fractures
    Middle fossa basilar skull fractures (across mastoid air cells, middle ear, etc.)
    Penetrating head injuries
  Postoperative (neurosurgical)
  Infections of the face or scalp
  Dental infections
  Congenital anomalies of the skull (e.g., encephaloceles)
Hematogenous spread
  Cyanotic heart disease
    Right-to-left shunts
    Valvular disease
    Septal defects
  Lung disease
    Bronchiectasis
    Lung abscess or empyema
    Rarely, cystic fibrosis
    IV drug abuse
    Other distant focus of infection
Immunosuppression
  Steroids
  Antimetabolite therapy
  Congenital immunodeficiency disorders
  Acquired immunodeficiency syndrome
Neonates
Sickle cell disease
Congenital CNS malformations
  Dysraphic sites (myelomeningoceles, neurenteric cysts, etc.)
  Sinus tracts associated with dermoids, etc.

Brain abscesses present initially with poorly localizable and vague neurologic complaints. Dull headache and low grade fever associated with predisposing factors are sufficient to clinically raise the suspicion of an intracranial suppurative process. Typical clinical signs and symptoms of brain abscess vary with the localization of the abscess.

TABLE 13-2. SIGNS AND SYMPTOMS OF BRAIN ABSCESS

Headache
   Poorly localizable
   Dull
   Worsened by Valsalva maneuver or position change
Fever
   Prolonged course
   Absent in 30-50% of cases
Expanding mass and increased intracranial pressure
   Vomiting
   Somnolence, confusion
   Papilledema late and present in less than 50% of cases
   Focal signs: aphasia, hemiparesis, ataxia, lower cranial nerve
    findings
   Presentations may be either insidious or "stroke-like"

The present availability of CT and NMR has dramatically changed the time frame in which brain abscesses are diagnosed and treated. Initial nonbacteriologic confirmation and longitudinal follow-up on empiric therapy can be directed with serial CT scans. Frequent reports now indicate that "ring enhancement" seen on CT does not necessarily correlate with surgical encapsulation. Focal areas of edema of the cerebral or cerebellar cortex may appear on CT days before enhancement becomes evident. Periabscess edema frequently produces significant mass affect. CT and NMR allow accurate localization of abscesses for neurosurgical procedures including open or needle drainage and permit noninvasive evaluation of the clinical course.

Lumbar Puncture

Lumbar puncture may be significantly hazardous in patients with brain abscesses or other focal mass lesions. Increased intracranial pressure with focal masses may produce tangential forces that herniate brain tissue across fixed structures such as the tentorium cerebelli or other dural surfaces when lumbar puncture is performed and spinal fluid removed. In most cases of unruptured brain abscesses, CSF examination does not contribute significantly to the diagnosis. Frequently, few or no inflammatory cells are present. Cultures of the CSF often do not reveal any microorganisms. The opening pressure at the time of lumbar puncture may be significantly elevated and suggest a medical emergency.

Radiographs of the Skull

Radiographs of the skull in pediatrics contribute very little to the diagnosis of the brain abscess. Occasionally sinusitis may be detected in the frontal, ethmoid, or sphenoid sinuses. Evidence of mastoiditis may be present on views. Because the pineal gland is not often calcified in children, mass shifts across the dura may not be detected.

Echoencephalography, Brain Scans, and Electroencephalography

Echoencephalography and brain scans have very little or no usefulness currently in the diagnosis and management of brain abscess. Although electroencephalography may aid in the localization of abscess, this task should be reserved exclusively for CT or NMR.

Other studies to be considered in detecting the source of hematogenous spread contributing to brain abscess should include echocardiography for evidence of valvular defects or vegetations. Although the CBC is routinely done, it contributes little to the clinical impression of brain abscess. Blood cultures both for aerobic and anaerobic bacterial and fungal agents such as nocardia, candida, and other fungal organisms should be obtained, particularly when valvular heart disease and right-to-left shunts are present.

Treatment. Early diagnosis and medical management of brain abscess and other intracranial suppurative lesions are now possible with CT. For this reason the criteria for surgical intervention are controversial. The stage of brain abscess encapsulation, amount of edema and mass affect on CT, and the general medical state of the patient often determine which general treatment option is followed.

TABLE 13–3. GENERAL TREATMENT OPTIONS IN BRAIN ABSCESS MANAGEMENT

IV broad spectrum antibiotic therapy for several days to 2 wk followed by surgical excision of the encapsulated brain abscess

Needle aspiration of the encapsulated abscess and appropriate IV antibiotic therapy determined by cultures of the exudate

Aspiration followed by complete excision and appropriate IV antibiotics

Medical management alone with broad spectrum intravenous antibiotics without surgical intervention unless clinical or CT evidence of deterioration occurs.

TABLE 13–4. BACTERIAL ORGANISMS CAUSING BRAIN ABSCESS

Common causes
  Anaerobes
  Staphylococcus aureus
  Streptococcus pyogenes
  Streptococcus viridans
  Streptococcus pneumoniae
Less common causes
  Citrobacter sp.
  Enterobacter sp.
  Klebsiella sp.

(continued)

TABLE 13-4. (continued)

Escherichia coli
Proteus sp.
Pseudomonas sp.
Hemophilus sp.
Nocardia sp.
Listeria monocytogenes

TABLE 13-5. MEDICAL AND SURGICAL MANAGEMENT
OF BRAIN ABSCESS

For suspected anaerobes
  Chloramphenicol 100 mg/kg/day div q6h
For *Staphylococcus aureus*
  Vancomycin 40 mg/kg/day IV div q6h *OR* nafcillin 200-400
  mg/kg/day div q6h
For coliform bacilli infections
  Moxalactam or cefotaxime 200 mg/kg/day IV div q6h *OR*
  ceftriaxone 100 mg/kg/day div q12h
  OR ampicillin 400 mg/kg/day div q6h and chloramphenicol 100
  mg/kg/day div q6h
  Duration of therapy: minimum 21 days

FUNGAL INFECTIONS

Fungal infections of the CNS may account for both acute and
subacute deteriorations in neurologic function, particularly in
children with factors predisposing them to opportunistic infections. Even with a high index of clinical suspicion, the diagnosis
of fungal infection is frequently delayed.

TABLE 13-6. FACTORS PREDISPOSING CHILDREN TO
FUNGAL CNS INFECTIONS

Primary immunodeficiency
Secondary immunodeficiency
  Corticosteroid therapy

TABLE 13-6. (continued)

Antimetabolite therapy (e.g., azothioprine)
Cytotoxic therapy (e.g., cyclophosphamide)
AIDS
Chronic disease
  Diabetes mellitus
  Leukemia or lymphoma
  Chronic renal disease
  Cystic fibrosis
Organ transplantation
IV therapy or drug abuse
Hematogenous spread from other foci
  Cardiac valvular disease
  Primary pulmonary fungal disease
  Primary cutaneous fungal disease
Contiguous spread
  Orbital, sinus, or cutaneous spread (e.g., mucormycosis)

Insidious changes in neurologic function, such as unexplained lethargy, psychosis, or irritability, may be the earliest symptoms of fungal infection. More alarming features, including focal or generalized seizures, meningismus, single or multiple cranial neuropathies, hemiparesis, and papilledema, occur as fungal diseases progress in the brain. It is crucial that patients be diagnosed early, in part, because of preexisting and debilitating disorders and, in part, because of prolonged therapy with relatively toxic agents required following diagnosis. Emphasis must be placed on a high clinical index of suspicion.

TABLE 13-7. DIAGNOSTIC APPROACH TO FUNGAL CNS INFECTIONS

Fungal cultures
  CSF
  Blood
  Sputum
  Tissue aspirates

(continued)

TABLE 13-7. (continued)

CSF analysis
    Cell count
    Glucose
    Protein
    Culture: large amounts of CSF are required
    Special stains, e.g., India ink
    Immunoglobulin electrophoresis or oligoclonal banding
Serum serologic assays
Tissue biopsy for histology and culture
    Meninges
    Brain
    Skin
    Lung

The typical pathologic patterns of fungal CNS infections accounting for the evolution of signs and symptoms in these disorders are quite variable and usually subtle.

TABLE 13-8. TISSUE REACTIONS TO FUNGAL INFECTIONS

Meningitis: acute, subacute, or chronic
Meningoencephalitis
Abscess: solitary, multiple, microabscesses
Granulomas
Arterial thrombosis

The number of specific fungal organisms associated with CNS infections are numerous. Only in unusual circumstances, e.g., mucormycosis, in which orbital and sinus complications are prominent, are characteristic features noted.

TABLE 13-9. FUNGAL ORGANISMS ASSOCIATED WITH CNS INFECTION

Histoplasma capsulatum—histoplasmosis
Coccidioides immitis—coccidioidomycosis
Blastomyces dermatitidis—North American blastomycosis
Aspergillus fumigatus—asperigillosis
Candida albicans—candidiasis
Cryptococcus neoformans—cryptococcosis (torulosis)
Rhizopus sp.—mucormycosis
Allescheria boydii—madurosporosis
Sporothrix schenkii—sporotrichosis
Nocardia asteroides—nocardiosis

The treatment of fungal infections of the CNS is crucially dependent on early recognition and the alleviation of predisposing factors. The most widely used antifungal agents are amphotericin B, 5-flucytosine, and miconazole.

Amphotericin B when used intravenously must be diluted with 5% dextrose to a concentration no greater than 1 mg per 10 ml and given as a 4- to 6-hour infusion. Amphotericin B is highly nephrotoxic and has limited CNS penetration when used systemically. For that reason, intrathecally administered amphotericin B is often used, particularly in coccidioidal infections. Added CNS toxicity occurs with intrathecal administration.

When administered orally, 5-flucytosine, has excellent penetration into the CNS. The role of 5-flucytosine remains controversial, however, and generally is used in combination with amphotericin B in patients with moderate to severe fungal CNS infections.

Miconazole, a recent antifungal agent, has selected indications in sensitive fungal invasive infections such as histoplasmosis, cryptococcosis, and candidiasis. It may be the drug of choice in certain fungal infections poorly responsive to amphotericin B, including Allescheria. In CNS infections, intrathecal administration of miconazole may be required because the agent has poor CNS penetration.

**TABLE 13-10. ANTIFUNGAL AGENTS FOR CNS
INFECTIONS: DRUG DOSAGES AND TOXICITIES**

Antifungal Agent	Dosage	Toxicity
Amphotericin B	IV: 0.6 to 1.0 mg/kg/day Duration: total dose 30 mg/kg	*Immediate*: chills, fever, nausea, vomiting Hypokalemia Phlebitis at injection site Normochromic, normocytic anemia Nephrotoxicity *Idiosyncratic*: anaphylactoid shock Hepatic failure Seizures Ventricular fibrillation
	Intrathecal: initial test dose of less than 0.1 mg in the adult to detect allergic effects followed by 0.25-0.50 mg mixed in 5 ml of distilled water or CSF given every other day	Pain in back and legs Aseptic meningitis Arachnoiditis Systemic toxicities from absorption from CSF
5-Flucytosine	Oral: 100-150 mg/kg/day in four divided doses to maintain serum level of 60-80 μg/ml	Bone marrow suppression Aplastic anemia Diarrhea Psychosis Hepatic dysfunction

Symptomatic care of children with CNS fungal infections includes evaluation clinically and by laboratory for the syndrome
of inappropriate ADH, insidiously developing hydrocephalus,

and thrombotic infarctions. Seizures frequently occur and require therapy adapted to impaired renal and hepatic function.

VENTRICULITIS (SHUNT INFECTION)

Shunt obstruction and infection are the most frequent and serious complications following placement of ventriculoperitoneal shunts. As many as 20 to 40% of the shunts ultimately become infected. In particular, neonates and young infants appear highly susceptible. There may also be an increased incidence of ventriculitis in children with hydrocephalus associated with myelomeningoceles (Arnold-Chiari malformation). The presence of intracranial infection or bacteremia are absolute contraindications to initial shunt placement and frequently neurosurgeons consider any infection, including otitis media, a relative contraindication. In particular, prolonged operative time for shunt placement appears to correlate best with the risk of infection.

Immediately following shunt placement and for the first 1 to 2 months postoperatively, the risk of shunt infection is highest. Skin contamination is the likely source of colonization of the shunt. For this reason, by far the most common cause of infection is *S. epidermidis* or less commonly, *S. aureus*, diphtheroids, and fungal organisms, in particular *Candida*. Occasionally gram-negative bacilli including *E. coli*, *Pseudomonas*, *Klebsiella*, and *Proteus* may occur. There appears to be an increased incidence of *H. influenzae* meningitis in children with shunts.

TABLE 13-11. BACTERIAL ORGANISMS ASSOCIATED WITH SHUNT INFECTIONS

Staphylococcus epidermidis
Staphylococcus aureus
Diphtheroids
Escherichia coli
Pseudomonas sp.
Klebsiella sp.
Proteus sp.
Haemophilus influenzae

Usually the clinical recognition of shunt infection is not difficult. Occasionally the operative incision may appear frankly purulent, erythematous and indurated. Fever, hypotension, or other clinical evidence of sepsis may be present in these cases. On the other hand, infection with *S. epidermidis* may appear more insidiously with only signs of local infection over the shunt incision site. Concomitantly, shunt obstruction with subacute decompensation suggests progressive hydrocephalus. Other findings are lethargy or irritability, papilledema, cranial nerve findings such as sixth nerve pareses or other oculomotor disturbances, and corticospinal tract dysfunction. Preexisting seizure disorders may worsen with the presence of shunt infection or obstruction.

The examination of CSF by shunt bulb aspiration is the most sensitive and safe procedure for documenting the etiology of shunt infection. Surgically prepping the site of the shunt bulb and using a small gauge needle (26-gauge) permits the aspiration of sufficient CSF for gram stain, bacterial and fungal cultures, chemistries, and cell count. Alternatively, lumbar puncture may be performed in those instances where decompensated hydrocephalus is not clinically suspected. The presence of increased intracranial pressure by examination of the skull, fundi, cranial nerves, or other aspects of the neurologic examination may suggest decompensated hydrocephalus in which lumbar puncture is contraindicated. Blood cultures should always be obtained. Other abnormal laboratory values may include a prominent leukocytosis.

The approach to the treatment of ventriculitis depends somewhat on the causative organism. Traditionally, high dose intravenous antibiotics combined with immediate shunt removal have been the treatment of choice. On occasion (approximately 15%), high dose IV antibiotics alone are sufficient. The combined approach of intrathecal and intraventricular antibiotics alone, or in combination with high dose intravenous antibiotics and shunt removal also occasionally have been reported to be successful with reduced neurologic morbidity and mortality.

The initial medical management of shunt infection includes IV vancomycin in doses of 40 mg/kg/day divided q6h pending the return of cultures. In particular, in cases of staphylococcal infection, an adherent and sticky layer of mucus may be embedded on the shunt tubing and prevent total sterilization of the ventricle and shunt system by IV antibiotics alone. In cases where after the first 48 hours of treatment, clinical or bacteriologic improvement is not achieved, it is recommended that IV antibiotics be combined with shunt removal. Antibiotic therapy at this point should be tailored to the specific culture results and bacteriologic sensitivities.

Prophylactic therapy for shunt infections should routinely be used, particularly in those patients most susceptible to infection such as neonates, those with the Arnold-Chiari malformation, or debilitated patients. Suggested prophylactic regimens include the use of antistaphylococcal agents such as methicillin or nafcillin in doses of 30 to 50 mg/kg given 2 hours preoperatively and then repeated postoperatively. Other suggested prophylactic regimens have included intravenous vancomycin preoperatively and IV rifampin preoperatively and postoperatively. No widespread consensus exists regarding recommendations of prophylactic antibiotic therapy. There is widespread agreement, however, that thorough skin preparation, reduced operative time, and other aspects of meticulous surgical care minimize the chance of wound and shunt infection.

TABLE 13–12. INTRAVENTRICULAR ANTIBIOTICS FOR SHUNT INFECTION

Antibiotic	Daily Dose (mg)
Amikacin	4–10
Ampicillin	10–25
Carbenicillin	25–40
Cephalothin	25–50
Chloramphenicol	25–50
Gentamicin	2–8
Kanamycin	4–10
Methicillin	25–100
Tobramycin	2–8
Vancomycin	20

TABLE 13-13. IV ANTIBIOTICS FOR SHUNT INFECTION

Staphylococcus epidermidis or *Staphylococcus aureus*
    Nafcillin 200-400 mg/kg/day div q6h
    Vancomycin 40 mg/kg/day div q6h (for nafcillin-resistant
      organisms)
Gram-negative coliforms
    Cefotaxime 200 mg/kg/day div q6h
    Ceftriaxone 100 mg/kg/day div q12h
    Moxalactam 200 mg/kg/day div q6h

Removal of the shunt may be necessary if prompt response to
    antimicrobial therapy is not obtained.

VIRAL DISEASE OF THE CNS

Viral and postviral neurologic diseases are frequent in pediatric
practice. Although the majority of these disorders are benign and
self-limited, notable exceptions occur, including herpes encephalitis, some equine encephalitides, postinfectious encephalomyelitis, Guillain-Barré syndrome, and Reye's syndrome.

Several viruses cause meningoencephalitis. Although most
viral meningoencephalitis appears clinically similar, seasonal occurrence and associated systemic signs and symptoms may suggest a specific viral cause. Equine encephalitis, a mosquito-borne
viral disease, typically occurs in the warm months whereas herpes
encephalitis is sporadic. The presence of gastrointestinal signs
and symptoms may suggest an enteroviral agent whereas upper or
lower respiratory tract infections may suggest adenovirus as a potential etiology. CNS infectious and postinfectious disorders may
occur with common childhood disorders, such as varicella.

TABLE 13-14. VIRUSES ASSOCIATED WITH
MENINGOENCEPHALITIS

Arboviruses
    St. Louis encephalitis
    Western equine encephalitis
    Eastern equine encephalitis

TABLE 13-14. (continued)

California encephalitis
Japanese B equine encephalitis
Venezuelan equine encephalitis

Enteroviruses
  Polio types I, II, and III
  Coxsackie A and B
  Echo

Herpes viruses
  Herpes I and II
  Varicella-Zoster
  CMV
  Epstein-Barr

Miscellaneous
  Mumps
  Rubeola
  Adenovirus
  Influenza A, B
  Lymphocytic choriomeningitis virus

The clinical signs and symptoms of viral meningoencephalitis are dependent upon the age of the child, severity of illness, and to a lesser extent, the specific viral agent. In general, mental status changes ranging from coma to delirium, focal or generalized seizures, meningismus, and fever are typical presenting features. Diagnosis is usually confirmed by the examination of the CSF and the exclusion of other bacterial, protozoan, or fungal organisms. Exceptions to this rule are chemical meningoencephalitis and Mollaret's meningitis, the latter a disorder of recurrent aseptic meningitis of unknown etiology. Routine studies of the CSF include measurement of the opening pressure, cell count and differential, protein and glucose determination with comparison to the serum glucose level, and viral, bacterial, and fungal cultures when appropriate. Gram stain of the CSF should be carefully examined. The presence of gross or microscopic blood in the CSF suggests the possibility of herpes or equine encephalitis.

Suspicion of herpes encephalitis is heightened by focal seizure activity, hemorrhagic CSF, and a fulminant course over several hours. Electroencephalography often reveals focal epileptiform activity and evidence of tissue destruction. CT scans may be notoriously misleading early in the course of herpes encephalitis. Despite strong clinical suspicion and focal epileptiform activity on EEG, the CT may remain normal for several days into the clinical course. The CT eventually reveals focal edema and possible hemorrhage in unilateral or bilateral temporal and orbitofrontal regions of the brain. Confirmation of herpes encephalitis requires viral growth on cultures, positive fluorescent antibody stains of biopsied brain tissue, or a fourfold rise of antibody titer documented between acute and convalescent specimens. Brain biopsy of suspected herpes encephalitis, although useful in confirming the diagnosis, may be hazardous in some settings.

In general, the treatment of viral meningoencephalitis involves supportive management, whether the patient is hospitalized or followed at home. Analgesics, in selected cases, and fluid and electrolyte therapy are usually sufficient. More fulminant cases of viral meningoencephalitis, in particular herpes encephalitis, may rapidly progress and leave the child with severe morbidity or death. The treatment of herpes encephalitis is acyclovir 30 mg/kg/day divided q8h IV for 10 days. The use of adenine arabinoside requires a significant amount of fluid to maintain drug solubility and may worsen some cases of focal cerebral edema associated with the viral encephalitis.

TABLE 13–15. POSSIBLE COMPLICATIONS OF VIRAL MENINGOENCEPHALITIS

Acute development of the syndrome of inappropriate ADH
Vomiting and dehydration
Seizure disorder
Behavior disturbances: hyperactivity, delirium, attention deficits

---

Postviral disorders of the CNS are not rare. Reye's syndrome and Guillain-Barré syndrome are discussed in Chapter 1. Postviral encephalomyelitis may occur in children recovering from common viral illnesses. The presence of signs and symptoms of optic neuritis, focal seizure activity, myelitis, ataxia, and other motor disturbances such as hemiparesis, monoparesis, or paraparesis suggests this neurologic disorder. The chronologic progression of postviral encephalitis may be insidious or fulminant. In addition to the studies used for the evaluation of acute meningoencephalitis, cerebrospinal immunoglobulin electrophoresis, and oligoclonal banding is useful. CT scan, EEG, and the assessment of visual, auditory, and spinal pathways by evoked potentials permit adequate localization and documentation of multiple lesions in the neuroaxis. Boluses of steroids, dexamethasone 2 mg/kg/day divided q6h IV (loading dose 2 mg/kg) appear useful, particularly for patients in whom visual and spinal cord integrity appears threatened.

Surgical Infections

Despite advances in virtually all aspects of both pediatric and surgical care, infection remains a major cause of morbidity and mortality in the pediatric surgical patient. Infection is one of the more common indications for operative intervention and also complicates the postoperative recovery of a significant number of children. Although no substitute for timely diagnosis, perioperative asepsis or meticulous technique, judicious use of antimicrobial therapy can greatly modify the postoperative course.

The role of antibiotics in surgery is seldom eradication of infection and, therefore, antimicrobial therapy is infrequently the sole treatment of choice for control of surgical infection. The unique nature of pediatric surgical sepsis usually dictates not only appropriate antimicrobial therapy but operative intervention to control infection. Proper use of antibiotics in this setting requires a thorough preliminary evaluation, familiarity with the signs and symptoms of the more commonly encountered infections, knowledge of the usual organisms involved, and timely operative intervention.

PROPHYLAXIS

Numerous factors have been identified that are directly related to the incidence of postoperative infection. Such factors include age and nutritional status of the patient, preliminary preparation of the operative site, length of the operative procedure, operative technique, and the use of blood and blood products. Most of these factors can be manipulated pre- or intraoperatively to minimize the incidence of postoperative infection. One factor, which cannot be manipulated by the surgeon, is the specific area of operative intervention. Certain operations have long been associated with unacceptably high rates of postoperative infection. Numerous studies in the adult surgical patient have demonstrated the efficacy of perioperative antimicrobial prophylaxis in diminishing postoperative infection. This principle has been applied to the pediatric surgical patient and now accounts for as much as 75% of the antibiotic use on pediatric surgical services. Unfortunately, it also accounts for the majority of cases of inappropriate antibiotic use in the same group. Effective prophylaxis is dependent upon adherence to specific guidelines of patient selection, choice of antibiotic, and timing and route of administration. Its use must be weighed against the risk of toxic or allergic reactions, emergence of drug-resistant strains and superinfection. Prophylaxis is, therefore, indicated only if the risk of infection outweighs these potential complications.

The risk of postoperative infection is related to the number of bacteria present in the operative field at the completion of the procedure. This in turn is dependent upon, among other things, the indication and specific operative procedure performed. These associations have resulted in the standardized classification of operative procedures by the U.S. Public Health Service.

TABLE 14-1. CLASSIFICATION OF OPERATIVE PROCEDURES

Clean
Nontraumatic
No inflammation
No break in technique
Respiratory, GU, GI tract not entered

Clean/Contaminated
Minor break in technique
Oropharynx entered
Respiratory or GI tract entered without significant spillage
Appendectomy
Biliary tract entered in the absence of infected bile
Vagina entered
GU tract entered in the absence of infected urine

Contaminated
Major break in technique
Fresh traumatic wound
Gross GI spillage
Biliary tract entered in the presence of infected bile
GU tract entered in the presence of infected urine

Dirty
Bacterial inflammation encountered
Transection of clean tissue for the purpose of access to purulence
Traumatic wound from "dirty" source
Traumatic wound with retained devitalized tissue, foreign body
  and/or fecal contamination
  Perforated viscus

Prophylactic antibiotics are not indicated in *clean* procedures unless the risk of infection is potentially life-threatening. Specific examples include cardiac surgery for structural defects, implantation of prosthetic material, or immunocompromised patients. Prophylaxis is indicated in those *clean/contaminated* cases where significant contamination is possible, such as biliary and colorectal surgery. Antibiotics are indicated in all *contaminated* and *dirty* cases and in most instances should be employed therapeutically rather than as prophylaxis.

Antibiotic selection for prophylaxis is based upon the usual sensitivity of the likely bacterial contaminant and no attempt should be made to cover all of the potential pathogens. Established efficacy, safety, physician familiarity, and cost should all be considered in the selection.

TABLE 14–2. RECOMMENDED PROPHYLACTIC ANTIBIOTICS

Procedure	Likely Contaminant	Antibiotic	IV Dose
Cardiovascular prosthetic implant	*Staphylococcus*	Cefazolin	50-100 mg/kg/day q6h
Biliary	Enteric gram-negative	Cefazolin	50-100 mg/kg/day q6h
Colorectal	Enteric gram-negative Anaerobic species	Cefoxitin	100 mg/kg/day q6h
Peritonitis/ ruptured viscus	Enteric gram-negative Enterococcus Anaerobic species	Gentamicin and ampicillin and clindamycin	7.5 mg/kg/day q8h 100 mg/kg/day q6h 40 mg/kg/day q6h
Traumatic	*Staphylococcus* *Streptococcus* *Clostridium*	Cefazolin	50-100 mg/kg/day q6h

Intravenous administration is the route of choice for antimicrobial prophylaxis. The drug should be administered so as to provide adequate tissue levels at the beginning of the operative procedure, usually within 1 hour of incision. Duration of therapy is controversial, but should not extend beyond 72 hours postoperatively. *Most children achieve maximum prophylaxis with a single preoperative and two postoperative dosages.*

WOUND INFECTIONS

The incidence of postoperative wound infection is directly related to the type (PHS classification) of operative procedure performed. Although wound infection occasionally results from exogenous contamination (e.g., normal skin flora, break in technique, poor site preparation), the incidence of this complication in clean cases should be less than 1%. Endogenous contamination accounts for the overwhelming majority of postoperative wound infections. Dirty cases have been associated with a 40% incidence of infectious complications. This can be avoided by alterations in usual techniques. Infection occurs in contaminated wounds closed primarily with the creation of subcutaneous dead space containing blood and necrotic tissue. Lack of skin and subcutaneous closure in these selected cases with subsequent delayed or secondary closure will avoid infectious complications.

Postoperative wound infection presents 4 to 14 days following operations. Clinical characteristics are dependent upon the organism involved. Staphylocccal infection appears from 4 to 7 days postoperatively and is associated with significant tenderness, erythema, and induration. Suppuration is prominent and purulent drainage may be apparent at the wound edges. Enteric gram-negative infection usually presents 7 to 14 days following surgery. Induration is present although erythema may be limited. Suppuration is less prominent and the drainage is frequently of a seropurulent nature. Wound infection may be associated with fever and leukocytosis, but systemic toxicity is more frequent with gram-negative infection. Suspicion of wound infection should prompt removal of the sutures with gentle separation of the wound edges. If infection is confirmed, culture is obtained, the remaining sutures removed and the wound opened throughout its extent. Treatment consists of irrigation and debridement of the involved tissue with subsequent wound packing. Idophor impregnated gauze is utilized until the wound is clean, usually 48 to 72 hours, followed by saline wet to dry dressings to stimulate granulation and allow secondary closure. Systemic antimicrobial therapy is unnecessary except where there is associated systemic toxicity.

An exception to the above guidelines is the occasional wound infected by group A streptococci. This presents as significant, rapidly spreading erythema within 24 to 48 hours of the surgical procedure. Drainage, if present, is serous. Treatment consists of systemic antistreptococcal therapy (penicillin G 100,000 to 200,000 U/kg/day q6h or cefazolin 50 to 100 mg/kg/day q6h for 10 days). The wound is left intact unless significant suppuration occurs.

TABLE 14–3. CHARACTERISTICS OF WOUND INFECTION

Organism	Time	Signs	Rx
Streptococcus	1–2 days	Rapidly spreading erythema and cellulitis	Penicillin G
Staphylococcus	4–7 days	Tenderness, erythema, suppuration, purulent drainage	Wound debridement and packing
Enteric gram-negative	7-14 days	Induration, seropurulent drainage, systemic toxicity	Wound debridement and packing

BURNS

The loss of the normal cutaneous barrier in the burned child renders the patient constantly at risk for infection. Bacterial invasion can convert previously favorable wounds to full thickness loss and, more importantly, remains a major cause of mortality in the thermally injured child. Despite the constant threat of sepsis and the significant complications associated with it, inappropriate, random use of parenteral antimicrobials will rapidly select out highly resistant, virulent species ultimately contributing to the morbidity and mortality of these children rather than aiding their recovery. Proper therapy of the bacterial component of burn injury depends upon an understanding of the normal microbial flora of burns, principles of wound care, and constant bacterial surveillance. The cornerstone of proper therapy is fastidious wound care and topical antimicrobial agents.

TABLE 14-4. ANTIMICROBIAL THERAPY OF BURNS

	Minor	Major
Characteristics	> 2 yr 2-3 degree < 20% total surface area (TSA) No major involvement of face, perineum, hands, and/or feet	< 2 yr 2-3 degree > 20% TSA Major involvement of face, perineum, hands and/or feet
Prophylaxis	None	*Tetanus*: toxoid 0.5 ml if immunized; antiserum in absence of immunization Penicillin 50,000 U/kg/day div q6h × 72 hr for group A streptococci

(*continued*)

TABLE 14-4. (continued)

	Minor	Major
Wound	Debridement Daily wash and saline rinse	Debridement Daily cleansing by hand or hydrotherapy
Topical	Silver sulfadiazine	Silver sulfadiazine
Dressing	Open or occlusive	Occlusive
Surveillance	Frequent wound evaluation	Initial swab culture Daily wound evaluation Weekly and prn wound biopsy, quantitative culture, and blood culture
Indications for systemic treatment	Usually unnecessary	$>10^5$ organisms/ cm^2 of wound surface Positive blood culture Clinical sepsis
Systemic antobiotics	Usually unnecessary	Based on culture results Usual organisms: *Staphylococcus, Streptococcus, E. coli*, and *Pseudomonas*

CHEST INFECTIONS

Mediastinum

The mediastinum is the space within the thoracic cavity bounded by the sternum, medial aspect of the pleura, and vertebral column. Its major contents include the heart, great vessels, esophagus, and trachea. Suppurative infection within the mediastinum is uncommon but always potentially lethal due to the absence of anatomic barriers and tendency for rapid spread. It is usually the result of iatrogenic contamination or contiguous spread from the neck and/or tracheobronchial lymph nodes. Established infection requires surgical drainage as well as appropriate antimicrobial therapy. The most frequent organisms encountered are gram-positive aerobic and anaerobic cocci.

TABLE 14-5. SUPPURATIVE MEDIASTINITIS

Symptoms	Pain
	Dyspnea
	Tachycardia
	Fever
Radiographic signs	Mediastinal emphysema
	Widened mediastinum
	Mediastinal air fluid level
Common organisms	Gram-positive cocci
	Anaerobes
Empiric therapy	Cefazolin 100 mg/kg day div q6h
	Surgical drainage

Empyema

Empyema is, for the most part, a complication of primary pulmonary infection. Once frequent, this infection is increasingly less common due to aggressive medical management of bacterial pneumonia. The most frequent organisms encountered in potentially complicated pneumonia are *Staphylococcus, Haemophilus influenzae,* group A *Streptococcus,* and *S. pneumoniae.*

TABLE 14-6. PNEUMONIAS ASSOCIATED WITH EMPYEMA

	Staphylococcal	*H. influenzae*	**Streptococcal**
Age	< 1 yr	3 mo–3 yr	3–5 yr
X-ray	Patchy bronchopneumonia	Lobar pneumonia	Diffuse bronchopneumonia
			(continued)

TABLE 14-6. (continued)

	Staphylococcal	*H. influenzae*	Streptococcal
Rx	Penicillinase-resistant penicillin	Ceftriaxone Cefotaxime	Penicillin or Ceftriaxone

Pleural fluid may occur with each of these organisms and surgical intervention is based upon the characteristics of that fluid. Empyema begins as an exudative effusion, which progresses to become fibrinopurulent and finally organized. Initial management includes thoracentesis for evaluation of the effusion and culture. Effusion may be treated by thoracentesis and seldom progresses with appropriate antibiotic therapy. Rapid reaccumulation of effusion with respiratory distress or the presence of fibrinopurulent fluid is an indication for tube thoracostomy. This is usually the consequence of infection caused by *S. aureus*. Organization of the empyema requires thoracotomy with decortication, although this is rarely necessary.

TABLE 14-7. SURGICAL TREATMENT OF EMPYEMA

Characteristics	Rx
Exudative effusion	Thoracentesis
Fibrinopurulent (pus)	Tube thoracostomy
Organized	Thoracotomy/decortication

Pulmonary Abscess

Abscess formation within the lung is most frequently encountered in the immunosuppressed or chronically ill child. Abscess may arise secondary to pneumonia, usually staphylococcal and/or *Klebsiella*, or as the result of aspiration of infected material containing anaerobic organisms. Selection of antibiotics should be guided by blood or lung aspirate cultures and should be continued for 3 to 6 weeks. Penicillin G is the appropriate antibiotic for anaerobic aspiration. With proper therapy, a gradual dissolution of the abscess cavity will be seen.

Surgical intervention may include bronchoscopy for culture or occasional transbronchial drainage. Thoracotomy and resection is reserved for chronic thick-walled abscesses, failure of medical management, or repeated infection.

GASTROINTESTINAL

Acute Abdomen

The majority of surgical infections involve the peritoneal cavity and the gastrointestinal organs. The various peritoneal membranes serve as semipermeable barriers and participate in the exchange of water and solutes. There is normally a small amount of clear, sterile fluid in the peritoneal cavity circulating in a defined fashion, bathing the intraabdominal structures. The quantity and quality of this fluid can change rapidly with alteration in hepatic, renal, or cardiovascular function as well as with various states of inflammation.

Infection and/or contamination within the peritoneal cavity results in inflammation of the lining with the outpouring of fluid and inflammatory cells. Although rarely effective in the dissolution of infection, this response can be highly effective in localizing the focus of involvement with resultant abscess formation.

Generalized peritonitis, regardless of the cause, presents with characteristic findings. Pain is the most constant symptom and is diffuse to both palpation and rebound. The child will resist efforts at movement. Abdominal rigidity is prominent and bowel sounds are absent. There may be severe toxicity and dehydration due to bacteremia and the intraabdominal loss of fluid. *Recognition of generalized peritonitis and appropriate resuscitation are paramount to efforts at determining etiology.* Once resuscitation has begun, broad spectrum antimicrobials are administered.

Peritonitis in the child is almost invariably the result of intestinal contamination. Specific common causes include ruptured appendicitis, closed loop intestinal obstruction, and perforated bowel. Although the enteric flora consists of a large number of potential pathogens, *Escherichia coli*, enterococcus, and *Bacteriodes fragilis* far and away lead the list of organisms causing peritonitis. Based on this experience, the antimicrobial therapy of peritonitis includes gentamicin 7.5 mg/kg/day q8h, ampicillin 200 mg/kg/day q6h, and clindamycin 40 mg/kg/day q6h. These antimicrobials are administered preliminary to surgical exploration and continued for 7 to 14 days.

Appendicitis

Appendicitis is one of the most frequent surgical conditions of childhood. Despite this, it is commonly misdiagnosed and approximately 50% of pediatric cases receive attention only after perforation has occurred. This is the stage at which postoperative septic complications are significantly increased. Acute appendicitis is a diagnosis made by physical examination. The sine qua non is localized right lower quadrant peritonitis. The pain, although epigastric to midabdominal initially, will invariably localize in the right lower abdomen and become associated with tenderness and signs of peritoneal irritation. It is usually associated with anorexia, nausea, and/or vomiting. Fever, however, is quite variable. These findings by an experienced examiner should prompt appendectomy. Laboratory and radiographic data never confirm nor preclude appendicitis in a child.

Antibiotics assume an adjunctive role in the treatment of appendicitis. Bacterial contamination outside of the appendix is absent in simple appendicitis. With time and progression of the process there will be transmural migration of bacteria culminating in perforation and frank abscess formation. Antibiotics are not indicated in the therapy of simple appendicitis. The difficulty is in determining preoperatively the pathologic state of the appendix. As a general rule, therefore, all patients with presumed appendicitis are begun on preoperative antibiotics.

If the history and physical signs indicate uncomplicated appendicitis, cefoxitin is begun. A single dose is employed with simple appendicitis. When suppuration is present, the child receives an additional two postoperative doses. When complicated appendicitis, i.e., gangrenous, ruptured, and/or abscessed, is suspected, gentamicin, ampicillin, and clindamycin are begun preoperatively. These are continued for a minimum of 5 days and are discontinued only if the child has been afebrile for 48 hours.

TABLE 14-8. ANTIBIOTICS IN APPENDICITIS

Simple	Cefoxitin 100-150 mg/kg/day q6h	1 dose preoperatively
Suppurative	Cefoxitin 100-150 mg/kg/day q6h	1 preoperatively 2 postoperatively
Gangrenous, perforated or abscessed	Gentamicin 7.5 mg/kg/day q8h,	Minimum 5 days
	Ampicillin 200 mg/kg/day q6h and Clindamycin 40 mg/kg/day q6h	

Gastric/Small Bowel

Most authors consider the normal stomach to be sterile due to the acid environment. Acid-tolerant organisms have been cultured but are seldom pathogenic. Alterations in the stomach, its contents, or motility may result in significant bacterial colonization. Such alterations include previous pyloric or ulcer surgery, gastric bypass (gastrojejunostomy), and intestinal obstruction with secondary gastric alkalinization. Similarly, the upper small bowel is relatively "sterile" in its normal state with increasing bacterial colonization as one proceeds distally. A variety of gram-positive and gram-negative, aerobic and anaerobic organisms have been recovered. As one approaches the terminal ileum, the flora become more characteristic of the so-called "enteric" organisms, such as *E. coli*, enterococcus, and *Bacteroides*. Alteration in the normal small bowel flora are again related to abnormalities of motility and function as is seen following intestinal obstruction.

Antibiotic coverage in elective gastro/upper intestinal surgery is controversial. Antibiotics are not indicated in the elective case with little chance of contamination. In the presence of alteration of normal flora, high risk of contamination, or a compromised patient, prophylactic antibiotic coverage is indicated. The drug of choice is cefazolin, 100 mg/kg/day q6h.

Elective surgery in the distal small bowel is more likely to result in contamination with enteric flora. Antibiotic coverage is utilized prophylactically only according to the guidelines previously outlined. Cefoxitin, 100 to 150 mg/kg/day divided q6h, is indicated in these cases.

Neonatal Necrotizing Enterocolitis

Necrotizing enterocolitis (NEC) is an inflammatory septic process of the distal small bowel. It classically occurs in the "stressed" premature within the first week of life and usually involves the terminal ileum. Although the etiology remains unclear, it appears to result from ischemic injury to the bowel with subsequent enteric bacterial invasion. Although a number of microorganisms have been implicated, none have been consistently associated with NEC.

Affected newborns usually present with the nonspecific signs of sepsis (thermal lability, thrombocytopenia, gastric retention) as well as abdominal distention and occult blood in the stool (see Chap. 2). The sine qua non for diagnosis is the radiographic finding of pneumatosis intestinalis, i.e., air within the bowel wall. The initial management is nonoperative and includes correction of fluid and electrolyte abnormalities, gastric decompression, and gut "rest." Umbilical catheters should be removed. Broad spectrum antibiotics are employed. As the organisms involved are usually enteric, gentamicin, ampicillin, and clindamycin should be given initially. Therapy may then be modified based on culture results. Stool cultures are particularly helpful in isolating associated abnormal flora.

These infants must be monitored frequently and carefully for the development of both medical (e.g., shock and DIC) and surgical complications, e.g., intestinal gangrene, perforation, and obstruction. In the absence of these, therapy is continued for 7 to 10 days. If there are no recurrent symptoms 24 hours following cessation of antibiotics, feedings are resumed.

TABLE 14-9. NECROTIZING ENTEROCOLITIS

Signs	"Sepsis"
	Bilious aspirates
	Abdominal distention
	Heme + stool
X-ray	Pneumatosis intestinalis
Therapy	Correction of fluid and electrolyte abnormalities
	NPO
	Gastric decompression
	Parenteral antibiotics
Antibiotics	Gentamicin, ampicillin, and clindamycin for 7-10 days (for doses, see Table 18-10)
Complications	Intestinal gangrene
	Perforation
	Obstruction
	Shock
	DIC

Colon

The colon has the largest concentration of microorganisms of any structure within the peritoneal cavity. Initially sterile in the newborn, the large bowel becomes colonized by approximately 8 hours of life. Operations on the colon, therefore, have the potential for significant contamination. Bacterial counts can be reduced preoperatively by vigorous cleansing of the colon in elective cases. Nonabsorbable oral antibiotics have been extensively used preoperatively in the adult to reduce enteric flora counts. The preoperative maneuvers utilized in the adult have not been successful in the child. Strong cathartics and frequent enemas risk electrolyte and fluid abnormalities, particularly in the infant. The nonabsorbable antibiotics frequently result in emesis. Fecal bulk can, however, be reduced in elective pediatric cases by several days of clear liquids combined with a mild preoperative laxative such as milk of magnesia. Immediate preoperative irrigation, in the operating room, with a dilute povidone-iodine solution may also reduce bacterial counts. Prophylactic parenteral antibiotics are indicated in colon surgery in the child. Cefoxitin, 100 to 150 mg/kg/day, provides adequate coverage in elective cases. In those instances where preoperative preparation is impossible, gentamicin 7.5 mg/kg/day q8h, ampicillin 100 mg/kg/day q6h, and clindamycin 40 mg/kg/day q6h should be used prophylactically.

Anorectal

The anorectal region is uniquely resistant to infection. This may be due to the copious blood supply or the squamous epithelium. Operation in this area is seldom complicated by sepsis and few surgeons perform a formal preoperative "bowel prep" for elective cases. Prophylactic antibiotics are, however, frequently utilized, particularly in the young child. Cefoxitin, 100 to 150 mg/kg/day, covers the majority of organisms likely to be encountered.

Spontaneous infection in the anorectal region is encountered in the child. It usually occurs in the infant less than 2 years of age, and is caused by *S. aureus* and *E. coli* with equal frequency. The origin is similar to the adult, arising in the crypts of the dentate line with extension to the perirectal or perianal tissues. This usually presents as a small area of fluctuance surrounded by induration and erythema somewhere in the perianal region. Treatment consists of adequate surgical drainage. Antimicrobials are indicated when suppuration is associated with systemic toxicity or significant cellulitis (Chap. 4). These children must also be followed postoperatively to detect the occasional child who will develop a chronic perianal fistula.

Biliary

Biliary tract disease is uncommon in the pediatric population and is of two main types, postoperative biliary atresia and cholecystitis.

Bile drainage can now be surgically achieved in a significant percentage of children with biliary atresia. The exposure of the intrahepatic biliary system to the GI tract by creation of the hepatoportoenterostomy places these children at constant risk for cholangitis. Cholangitis, in turn, is a serious complication as it can result in complete cessation of bile flow in a previously successful case. Most such children are, therefore, maintained on bacterial suppression such as trimethoprim-sulfamethoxazole suspension, 4/20 mg/kg/day divided q12h, for a variable length of time. Unexplained fever in a postoperative biliary atresia patient must be presumed to represent cholangitis until proven otherwise. Other confirmatory signs include diminution of bile flow (if a diverting stoma is present) or a rise in the serum bilirubin. Treatment of suspected cholangitis is empirical, as bile in these children is colonized and usually contains a variety of enteric organisms, any one of which may be causative. Blood cultures are rarely positive. An aminoglycoside, such as gentamicin 7.5 mg/kg/day q8h, offers the widest coverage for the organisms encountered as well as providing high hepatic concentrations. Parenteral therapy is continued for a minimum of 5 days. Failure of response within 24 to 48 hours should prompt reevaluation of antibiotic coverage, as well as consideration of possible "mechanical" abnormalities in the biliary conduit itself.

TABLE 14-10. CHOLANGITIS IN BILIARY ATRESIA

Suppression	TMP-SMX suspension 4/20 mg/kg/day div q12h
Signs	Unexplained fever Leukocytosis ↓ bile flow ↑ serum bilirubin
Treatment	Gentamicin 7.5 mg/kg/day q8h for a minimum of 5 days

Symptomatic cholecystitis in childhood is classically associated with hemolytic disease, most frequently sickle cell anemia. It is rare to operate on these children acutely and, therefore, antibiotic therapy is used prophylactically. The drug of choice is cefazolin 100 mg/kg/day q6h.

Hepatic

Pyogenic liver infection is unusual in the child. It is most frequently encountered in the chronically ill or the immunosuppressed patient. Pylephlebitis, septicemia of the portal vein, secondary to ruptured appendicitis was historically considered the most common etiology. Although infrequent today, this may still result in abscess formation. Similarly, liver abscess may rarely arise in the newborn period due to umbilical vein catheterization. Other causes of liver abscess include septicemia with hepatic seeding, cholangitis, and bacterial contamination of preexisting cystic disease of the liver.

Liver involvement may be diffuse "microabscess" formation or single to multiple "macro" abscesses. No single bacterium predominates and the abscess may contain multiple species. Grampositive, gram-negative, and anaerobic species both singly and together have been reported. Symptoms are nonspecific, those of sepsis, and rarely characteristic of hepatic pathology. Liver abscess should, therefore, be considered in the chronically ill child with evidence of ongoing sepsis of unknown etiology. Diagnosis is facilitated by sonography and hepatic scintiscan. Therapy is initially intensive broad spectrum antibiotics with subsequent alteration in coverage based on culture results. Macroabscess lends itself to surgical drainage, which may occasionally be performed percutaneously. Drainage is not possible with diffuse microabscess formation.

POSTOPERATIVE FEVER

One of the most frequent problems encountered on a pediatric surgical service is evaluation of a child with postoperative fever. Thorough physical examination is mandatory and always precedes laboratory and radiographic evaluation. Cultures are frequently unnecessary and antibiotic therapy is seldom indicated.

The likely causes of fever in the postoperative child are directly related to the time elapsed following surgery and are almost always detectable by thoughtful examination. It must also be remembered that hospitalization does not exclude the patient from the normal diseases of childhood.

Fever in the immediate postoperative period usually accompanies surgery for septic processes. Manipulation of the infected area (e.g., ruptured appendix) results in bacteremia with a febrile response. This response is transient and requires no specific therapy other than the appropriate preoperative selection of antibiotics, adequate fluid resuscitation, and occasional antipyretics.

Fever appearing within the first 24 hours of operation almost invariably is the result of atelectasis. Postoperative pain leads to the withholding of cough and shallow respirations. This, in turn, results in areas of atelectasis in the dependent portions of the lung with a secondary febrile response. The exact mechanism of fever in this process is controversial. The fever is usually low grade. Auscultation demonstrates diminished breath sounds in the lung base and rhonchi. Management consists of adequate analgesia without respiratory depression, early postoperative mobilization, and occasional respiratory therapy such as percussion, postural drainage, and incentive spirometry. In difficult cases, nasotracheal suction may be required. Failure of management may lead to major segmental and/or lobar collapse requiring bronchoscopy for reinflation. Similarly, neglected atelectasis can lead to frank pneumonitis.

Over the subsequent 48 hours postoperatively, atelectasis remains prominent, but additional causes of fever should be considered. More common etiologies include: use of nasogastric intubation predisposing to otitis in the child, urinary tract infection secondary to instrumentation, and catheter-induced phlebitis. The wound must also be carefully examined for signs of streptococcal infection.

By 4 days postoperatively, the more common cause of fever is wound infection. This is detectable by close inspection of the operative site.

Intraabdominal abscess, although infrequent, may become

symptomatic by as early as 5 days postoperatively. It most frequently follows surgery for complicated appendicitis and the onset and signs are usually insidious in nature. There is frequently a postoperative period of improvement with subsequent recrudescence of fever and leukocytosis. Localized pain and tenderness may be present. Other signs and symptoms vary with location, such as pleural effusion with subphrenic abscess, ileus or obstruction with intraloop abscess, and diarrhea with pelvic abscess. Physical examination, plain radiographs, and ultrasonography are most helpful in localizing the abscess. Treatment is surgical drainage. Although intraabdominal abscesses must be considered as the cause of fever in the late postoperative period, it is unusual and less likely than the etiologies previously enumerated.

TABLE 14-11. POSTOPERATIVE FEVER

Time	Common Etiology
Immediate	Operative manipulaton of infected area
Day 1	Atelectasis
Day 2–3	Atelectasis
	Otitis media
	Phlebitis
	Urinary tract
	Streptococcal wound
Day 4	Wound
	Otitis media
	Phlebitis
	Urinary tract
Day 5–beyond	Wound
	Otitis media
	Phlebitis
	Urinary tract
	Intraabdominal abscess

Sexually Transmitted Diseases

The five classic venereal diseases (gonorrhea, syphilis, chancroid, lymphogranuloma venereum, and granuloma inguinale) have been joined by the most prevalent sexually transmitted disease (STD) in the United States, *Chlamydia trachomatis* and other common STD-associated syndromes. These diseases can be classified on the basis of etiology or clinical manifestations.

TABLE 15-1. STD ETIOLOGIES

Type	Disease
Bacterial	
Neisseria gonorrhoeae	Urethritis, cervicitis, PID, perihepatitis, disseminated/sepsis, proctitis
Treponema pallidum	Congenital, primary/secondary syphilis
Chlamydia trachomatis	Urethritis, cervicitis, PID, perihepatitis, proctitis, conjunctivitis-pneumonitis
non-trachomatis	Lymphogranuloma venereum
Ureaplasma urealyticum	Urethritis, cervicitis, endometritis (postpartum fever)
Gardnerella vaginalis	Nonspecific vaginitis
Haemophilus ducreyi	Chancroid
Calymmatobacterium granulomatis	Granuloma inguinale
Shigella	Shigellosis (homosexual males)
Group B streptococci	Neonatal sepsis/meningitis
Viral	
HSV	Initial and recurrent genital herpes, meningitis, meningoencephalitis, neonatal herpes, cervical carcinoma
Hepatitis B	Acute hepatitis, chronic active or persistent hepatitis, polyarteritis nodosa, hepatoma
CMV	Heterophil-negative mononucleosis, congenital infection, cervicitis
Genital wart virus	Condyloma acuminata, infant laryngeal papilloma
Molluscum contagiosum	Molluscum contagiosum (genital)
Protozoan	
Trichomonas vaginalis	Vaginitis
Fungal	
Candida albicans	Vulvovaginitis, balanitis
Parasite	
Phthirius pubis	Pubic lice
Sarcoptes scabiei	Scabies

TABLE 15-2. CLINICAL MANIFESTATIONS

Syndrome	Etiology
Male urethritis	GC, chlamydia, HSV, ureaplasma
Genital ulceration	HSV, syphilis, chancroid, granuloma inguinale, LGV
Female lower GU tract infection	
Urethritis	GC, chlamydia
Vulvitis	Candida, HSV
Vaginitis	Trichomonas, candida, *G. vaginalis,*
Cervicitis	*M. hominis,* GC, chlamydia, HSV
Cervicitis with vaginitis	Candida, trichomonas
PID	GC, chlamydia, anaerobic bacteria, *M. hominis,* facultative gram-negative rods (*E. coli*), *Actinomyces israelii*
Proctitis	GC, chlamydia, HSV, ameba, hepatitis B, enteric bacteria, giardia
Acute arthritis with genital infection	GC (arthritis-dermatitis syndrome), chlamydia (Reiter's syndrome)
Infertility	
Postabortion, postsalpingitis	GC, chlamydia, *M. hominis*
Spontaneous abortion	HSV, GC, chlamydia

APPROACH TO STD

A careful history and complete physical examination are vital; in postmenarchal, sexually active females this should include a pelvic (speculum and bimanual) examination with a Pap smear. In a premenarchal child or adolescent with an intact hymen (suspect sexual abuse), an external examination in the frog-leg position allows visual inspection past the introitus. The history should help classify the STD and guide the physical examination. Important historical points include history of past STDs, last menstrual period, pregnancy, past history of UTIs, contraceptive methods or devices, sexual contacts (vital for their treatment), homosexual activity (as applicable), type of sexual activity (according to complaint—pharyngitis, proctitis, etc.), and last sexual activity.

Male Urethritis

Urethritis in males is suggested in any sexually active individual with dysuria and a discharge. The etiologic diagnosis of urethritis in males can be confirmed by gram stain; the most important objective is to confirm urethritis by examining for exudate in a urethrogenital swab taken 1 to 2 cm within the urethra. It is preferable to obtain a specimen in the morning prior to voiding. Gram stain smear containing greater than 5 WBC per 1000 × field suggests urethritis.

TABLE 15–3. GC VERSUS NGU OR HSV URETHRITIS

	GC	NGU[a]	HSV
Incubation (days)	2–7	14–21	2–7
Discharge	Profuse, yellow	Seen on arising or urethral stripping, white	Variable, mucoid
Dysuria	Moderate	Mild	Severe
Inguinal adenopathy	No	No	Yes
Penile lesions	No	No	Usually present
Gram stain	Gram-negative diplococci in neutrophils	Negative	Penile lesions, Tzanck positive

[a] 40-50% of NGU is due to chlamydia; *Ureaplasma urealyticum* has been implicated in chlamydia-negative cases.

The diagnosis of urethritis should exclude alternative diagnoses: epididymitis, arthritis-dermatitis syndrome, Reiter's syndrome, and prostatitis. The clinician must exclude prostatitis and cystitis in males with dysuria.

Acute Epididymo-orchitis

Acute epididymo-orchitis is almost always unilateral with a tender scrotum on palpation. This entity may be seen with or without fever. The differential diagnosis includes testicular torsion (surgical emergency), tumor (including leukemia relapse), and trauma. The etiologies are commonly GC or chlamydia and are usually associated with urethral discharge. A gram stain and/or culture of the discharge (GC or *chlamydia*) is indicated, and therapy includes bed rest, scrotal elevation, and antimicrobial therapy (see Treatment, Table 15-6).

Lower Genital Tract Infections in Females

The common symptoms of dysuria (burning), dyspareunia (painful sexual intercourse), vulvar irritation, and vaginal discharge are seen in lower genital tract infections in females.

TABLE 15-4. SYMPTOMS BY DISEASE

Urethritis
  Internal
    Dysuria (must exclude cystitis and vaginitis)
    Cystitis (UTI): bacteriuria ($\geq 10^5$/ml urine)
  External
    Acute urethral syndrome
      Dysuria and no evidence of bacteriuria (≥ 10 WBC per 400 $\times$ field and 10^2-10^4 bacteria/ml urine)
      GC or chlamydia possible etiologies (negative *unspun* urine gram stain)
  Cervicitis
    Vaginal discharge, exclude cervical ectopy (pregnancy and PO contraceptives), perineal syndrome (internal dysuria, bartholinitis, proctitis); associated PID
Vulvovaginitis
  Malodor, external dysuria, vaginal discharge, vulvar lesions (see Chap. 11)

Acute Pelvic Inflammatory Disease (PID)

The spectrum of acute PID includes endometritis, salpingitis, parametritis, and/or peritonitis. The symptoms of PID are lower abdominal pain and tenderness, bilateral adnexal tenderness on cervical motion, a recent onset vaginal discharge, and/or abnormal menstrual bleeding. The associated signs, symptoms, and laboratory abnormalities frequently include fever, chills, nausea, vomiting, adnexal mass, leukocytosis, elevated ESR, and history of previous PID episodes. If an IUD is present, there is a two- to ninefold increased risk, which is at a maximum during the first 2 months postinsertion.

The diagnosis of an adnexal mass is aided by a pelvic ultrasonography to exclude a tubo-ovarian abscess. Hospitalization for inpatient therapy is indicated under the following circumstances: diagnosis is unclear; pelvic abscess is suspected; patient is pregnant; outpatient therapy has failed, illness is severe; follow-up (after 48 to 72 hours) cannot be assured, and appendicitis or ectopic pregnancy cannot be excluded.

The complications of PID include infertility, recurrent PID, and ectopic pregnancy.

Genital Ulcer—Adenopathy Syndromes

Most genital ulcers cannot be diagnosed clinically, but thorough history and physical examination with simple diagnostic tests can be confirmatory.

TABLE 15–5. CLINICAL MANIFESTATIONS AND DIAGNOSTIC TESTS

	Incubation (days)	Ulcer	Nodes	Diagnosis
HSV	2–7	Painful, soft	Firm, tender	Tzanck preparation of vesicle or ulcer, fluorescent antibody, culture

TABLE 15-5. (continued)

	Incubation (days)	Ulcer	Nodes	Diagnosis
Syphilis	10–90	Painless, hard	Firm, nontender	Serology, dark-field of lesion
Chancroid	1–14	Painful, soft	Tender, fluctuant	Culture (newer selective enrichment media)
Granuloma inguinale	8–84 ($\curlywedge$ 30)	Painless, chronic spreading	Normal	Punch biopsy, histology (Donovan bodies)
LGV	3–21	Usually absent	Fluctuant, tender	Serology, isolation from node ($\curlywedge$ 30%)

In the evaluation of typical painful herpetic vesicopustules/ulcers, first, exclude syphilis by serology testing and then obtain a Tzanck preparation (positive in approximately 50% of properly collected smears) and/or culture ($\geq$ 90% positive). In painful nonvesicular ulcer(s) i.e. HSV versus chancroid, the lesions and/or inguinal nodes are painful. Isolation of HSV or *Haemophilus ducreyi* and syphilis serology are indicated.

In the diagnosis of painless ulcers use dark-field examination, and if available, serology. If negative and no other diagnosis is confirmed, then repeat serology 1 and 6 weeks later. For patients without improvement or who deteriorate over 1 to 2 weeks and diagnosis is still unknown, cultures for *H. ducreyi* and granuloma inguinale should be considered. Syphilis serology should be performed in all cases of genital ulcers.

TREATMENT

Following the clinical diagnosis of the disease entity (urethritis, PID), therapy should be tailored to all potential pathogens (empiric therapy) or to established diagnoses (Tables 15-6 through 15-11).

TABLE 15-6. GONORRHEA

Category	Treatment	Alternative Treatment and Other Considerations
Adults	Amoxicillin[a] 3.0 g Ampicillin[a] 3.5 g Aqueous procaine penicillin G[a] (APPG) 4.8 million U IM at 2 sites with probenecid 1 g Empiric therapy: up to 40-50% of GC patients have concomitant chlamydia infection; ampicillin/amoxicillin[a] (as above) *PLUS* tetracycline/doxycycline (as above)	Tetracycline 500 mg qid × 7 days Doxycycline hyclate 100 mg bid × 7 days Ceftriaxone 125 mg IM single dose
Older children	≥ 100 lb (45 kg) should receive adult regimens; < 100 lb (45 kg) single dose therapy—amoxicillin 50 mg/kg *PLUS* probenecid 25 mg/kg (1.0 g max), or aqueous procaine penicillin G[b] 100,000 U/kg IM plus probenecid	Penicillinase producing *N. gonorrhea* (PPNG): confirmed by culture and sensitivity testing, spectinomycin 40 mg/kg IM or ceftriaxone 125 mg IM Allergy to penicillin: spectinomycin (as above) or children with permanent teeth (generally over 8 yr), tetracycline 40 mg/kg day PO qid × 5 days

TABLE 15-6. (continued)

Category	Treatment	Alternative Treatment and Other Considerations
Complicated disease		
Disseminated; arthritis	Penicillin G 150,000 U/kg/day IV × 7 days	Cefotaxime 100 mg/kg/day IV qid × 7 days
Meningitis	Penicillin G 250,000 U/kg/day, IV in 6 divided doses × at least 10 days	Cefotaxime 200 mg/kg/day IV qid × at least 10 days or chloramphenicol 100 mg/kg/day IV qid × at least 10 days
Infants born to GC positive mothers (high risk)		
Full-term newborn	Aqueous crystalline penicillin G 50,000 U IM or IV; low birthweight newborns (prematures): aqueous crystalline penicillin G 20,000 U IM or IV	Topical ophthalmic prophylaxis should be offered but is not adequate treatment alone; clinical illness requires continuous therapy
Neonatal GC	Hospitalize, isolate for 24 hr posttreatment; aqueous crystalline penicillin G 50,000 U/kg/day IV bid × 7 days	Eyes irrigated immediately with saline or buffered ophthalmic solution and then hourly as long as necessary to eliminate discharge; topical therapy is not necessary with systemic therapy PPNG: ceftriaxone, cefotaxime or gentamicin

(*continued*)

TABLE 15–6. (continued)

Category	Treatment	Alternative Treatment and Other Considerations
	Complicated infection	
Disseminated arthritis	Aqueous crystalline penicillin G 75,000–100,000 U/kg/day IV qid × at least 7 days	
Meningitis	Aqueous crystalline penicillin G 100,000 U/kg/day IV tid or qid × at least 10 days	
PPNG	Spectinomycin 2.0 g (40 mg/kg) IM	Failure: cefoxitin 2.0 g IM plus probenecid 1.0 g; cefotaxime 1.0 g IM; trimethoprim/ sulfamethoxazole 9 tablets for 5 days (pharyngeal GC with PPNG)
Pregnancy	Amoxicillin/ampicillin with probenecid *PLUS* erythromycin 500 mg qid × 7 days (for chlamydia coverage)	Spectinomycin 2.0 g IM
DGI	Hospitalize; aqueous crystalline penicillin G 10 million U divided q4 or 6h IV qd until improvement, then amoxicillin tid (500 mg) or ampicillin (500 mg) qid PO to complete at least 7 days of therapy	Cefoxitin (1.0 g)/cefotaxime (500 mg), either IV qid × at least 7 days (treatment of choice for DGI due to PPNG), still consider concomitant chlamydia coverage; tetracycline (over age 8) 40 mg/kg qid PO × 7 days or erythromycin 50 mg/kg qid PO × 7 days

TABLE 15-6. (continued)

Category	Treatment	Alternative Treatment and Other Considerations
Secondary foci (DGI)		
Joints	Other than hips are not mandatory for open drainage; intraarticular antibiotics are not indicated	
Meningitis or endocarditis	High dose IV penicillin (as above); optimal duration unknown, minimum—1 mo	
Pharyngeal GC	APPG or tetracycline (as above); ampicillin/amoxicillin is inadequate	

[a] With probenecid 1 g.
[b] Preferred in proctitis/pharyngitis. Pediatric doses should not exceed adult doses.

Treatment for sexual partners should include an examination, culture, and treatment as described above (Table 15-6).

Ideally, follow-up cultures from infected sites should be done 4 to 7 days after treatment is completed. In women, rectal cultures for GC should be included.

For treatment failures, give spectinomycin 2.0 g (40 mg/kg) IM; if GC is recovered at failure, consider reinfection or PPNG (penicillinase producing *N. gonorrhoeae*). These GC isolates should be tested for penicillinase production. Benzathine penicillin G or PO penicillin are not recommended.

TABLE 15-7. CHLAMYDIA

Category	Treatment	Alternative Treatment and Other Considerations
Adult	Tetracycline HCL 500 mg PO qid × at least 7 days Doxycycline 100 mg PO bid × at least 7 days	Erythromycin 500 mg PO qid × at least 7 days
Older children (≤ 100 lb, ≤ 45 kg)	Tetracycline (permanent teeth, ≥ 8 yr) 10 mg/kg/day PO qid × 7 days; erythromycin (< 8 yrs, deciduous teeth) 40-50 mg/kg/day PO qid × 7 days	
During pregnancy (culture proven, unavailable or sexual partners have nongonococcal urethritis)	Erythromycin 500 mg PO qid on an empty stomach × at least 7 days	If regimen not tolerated 250 mg PO qid × 14 days (follow-up with cultures advised)
Established chlamydia conjunctivitis in infant	Erythromycin 40-50 mg/kg/day PO (as above) × at least 2 wk	Must rule out gonococcal involvement; nasal carriage important; topical therapy is of no additional benefit
Chlamydia pneumonia of infancy	Erythromycin therapy as above × at least 3 wk	

Examine and treat sexual partners. If available, posttreatment cultures are advisable as a follow-up. Cultures can be positive until 3 to 6 weeks after treatment. If they are positive, retreat.

TABLE 15-8. ACUTE PID

Category	Treatment	Alternative Treatment and Other Considerations
Hospitalize (if child ≤ 45 kg) then use dosing schedule per drug (Chap. 18)	Doxycycline 100 mg IV bid in combination with clindamycin 600 mg IV qid; *OR* cefoxitin 2.0 g IV qid; *OR* metronidazole 1.0 g IV bid (exclude pregnancy) *PLUS* gentamicin/tobramycin (in appropriate doses, Chap. 18) if facultative gram-negative rods isolated; IV for at least 4 days and at least 48 hr after patient defervesces. Then continue doxycycline 100 mg PO bid × 10-14 days of total therapy Patients may be followed with serial ultrasounds or physical examinations for response. If IUD present, an Ob/Gyn consultation for removal should be routine	
Ambulatory treatment (if child ≤ 45 kg) then use dosing schedule per drug (Chap. 18)	Amoxicillin 3.0 g PO; *OR* ampicillin 3.5 g PO; *OR* aqueous procaine penicillin G 4.8 million U IM, 2 sites; each regimen should include probenicid 1.0 g PO. Doxycycline 100 mg PO bid × 10–14 days) should be included in all adult regimens	Cefoxitin 2.0 g IM

No single agent is active against the entire spectrum of pathogens. Several combinations provide broad spectrum coverage in PID.

TABLE 15-9. ACUTE EPIDIDYMITIS

Category	Treatment	Alternative Treatment and Other Considerations
Older children (if child < 45 kg) then use dosing schedule per drug (Chap. 18)	Nongonococcal: tetracycline HCL 500 mg PO qid × at least 10 days. Doxycycline 100 mg PO bid × at least 10 days. GC: amoxicillin 500 mg PO tid × at least 10 days	Nongonococcal: erythromycin 500 mg PO qid × at least 10 days

Examine and treat sexual partners with regimen for uncomplicated GC and chlamydia infection.

Bed rest and scrotal elevation are recommended as a follow-up. Failure to improve over 2 to 3 days requires reevaluation and consideration of hospitalization. Reevaluation in 48 to 72 hours is mandatory; treatment failures should be hospitalized.

TABLE 15-10. FEMALE URETHRITIS AND CERVICITIS

Category	Treatment	Alternative Treatment and Other Considerations
Urethritis	See treatment GC, chlamydia	Urethral syndrome: $\geq$ 10 WBCs/400 × field, $10^2 - 10^4$ bacteria/ml urine, dysuria, frequency. Gram stain and/or culture—GC (treat as above for GC)

TABLE 15-10. (continued)

Category	Treatment	Alternative Treatment and Other Considerations
		Chlamydia proven or suspect (no bacteria)—treat as above for chlamydia Symptomatic and 10^2–10^4 bacteria (Gram stain unspun urine)—treat as acute urethral syndrome (Chap. 10)
Cervicitis	GC, chlamydia as above HSV: initial clinical episode, acyclovir, PO; IV (for severe constitutional symptoms, meningitis or immunocompromised host)—consult local expert	

TABLE 15-11. GENITAL ULCER/ADENOPATHY SYNDROMES

Category	Treatment	Alternative Treatment and Other Considerations
HSV (initial episode)	Acyclovir ointment—cover all lesions every 3 hr, 6 times a day × 7 days	Topical acyclovir can decrease duration of viral shedding and disease within 6 days of onset; it does *not* prevent recurrences *(continued)*

TABLE 15-11. (continued)

Category	Treatment	Alternative Treatment and Other Considerations
	Recurrent disease: no effective therapy for prevention or shortening disease; counseling and abstinence during prodrome or active lesions Oral acyclovir IV acyclovir—seldom appropriate in immunocompetent patients; if constitutional symptoms or lesions severe, consult local expert Follow-up: yearly Pap smear; use of condoms recommended by some but unproven	
Syphilis	(Child < 45 kg)	
Early (primary, secondary, latent of less than 1 yr)	Benzathine penicillin G: 2.4 million U IM	Penicillin allergic patient: tetracycline HC1 500 mg PO qid × 15 days
More than 1 yr duration (not neuro-syphilis)	Benzathine penicillin G: 2.4 million U IM 1 × wk for 3 successive wk	Penicillin allergic patient: tetracycline HC1 500 mg PO qid × 30 days
Neurosyph-ilis	Aqueous crystalline penicillin G: 12–24 million U IV per day	

TABLE 15-11. (continued)

Category	Treatment	Alternative Treatment and Other Considerations
	(2–4 million U q4h) × 10 days, then benzathine penicillin G: 2.4 million U IM weekly for 3 doses	
Pregnancy	Penicillin as in early syphilis regimen or more than 1 yr duration as appropriate	
Congenital	See categories below	Quantitative nontreponemal serology on infant and mother, treponemal serology results, history and physical examination then consult local expert for interpretation; CSF evaluation mandatory in confirmed cases
Symptomatic or asymptomatic with abnormal CSF	Aqueous crystalline penicillin G: 50,000 U/kg IM or IV daily in 2 divided doses for a minimum of 10 days	Aqueous procaine penicillin G: 50,000 U/kg, IM daily for a minimum of 10 days
Asymptomatic infants (normal CSF)	Benzathine penicillin G: 50,000 U/kg IM single dose	Follow-up: repeat quantitative nontreponemal tests at 3, 6, and 12 mo. Titers should drop to low titers or be nonreactive within a year. If neurosyphilis
Older children	Penicillin, same dosages as congenital syphilis but do not exceed adult dosage	

(continued)

TABLE 15–11. (continued)

Category	Treatment	Alternative Treatment and Other Considerations
		diagnosed and treated—follow-up at 6-mo intervals for 3 yr
		Retreatment: after repeat CSF evaluation; clinical signs/symptoms persist or recur; 4-fold increase in nontreponemal test; nontreponemal test initially high that fails to show a 4-fold decrease within 1 yr
		Sexual partners: exposed within 3 months or high risk epidemiologically—serology and treat
Chancroid	Erythromycin 500 mg PO qid × 10 days minimum and/or ulcers/lymph nodes heal	TMP/SMX: double strength tablet (160/800 mg) PO bid same duration
		Lesions: fluctuant lymph nodes should be aspirated through adjacent healthy skin; incision and drainage is contraindicated. Compresses can be applied to necrotic ulcers
		Sexual partners: treat as above for 10 days
		Nonresponders: antibiotic sensitivity testing on *H. ducreyi* recommended

TABLE 15-11. (continued)

Category	Treatment	Alternative Treatment and Other Considerations
Granuloma inguinale	Tetracycline 2 g qd × 10 days	Streptomycin 1 g IM bid × 10–15 days
LGV	Tetracycline 500 mg PO qid × at least 2 wk	Doxycycline 100 mg PO bid × at least 2 wk Lesions: fluctuant lymph nodes as for chancroid

MISCELLANEOUS INFECTIONS

Anogenital Warts, (Condylomata Acuminata)

If atypical or persistent warts are diagnosed they should be biopsied (linked to development of cancer). A Pap smear is recommended and therapy should be initiated only after results are known.

The therapy for external genital or perianal lesions is podophyllin 10 to 25% in compound tincture of benzoin. Apply to all warts and avoid normal tissues, follow by thorough washing in 1 to 4 hours. Podophyllin should be applied weekly for 4 weeks and if warts do not regress then alternative therapy should be considered. Alternative therapy can include cryotherapy, electrosurgery, or surgical removal. Cervical warts are treated effectively with cryotherapy. Vaginal warts as well as perianal warts, are eradicated with special attention to drying the lesions thoroughly before the speculum is removed. Anorectal or meatal warts should be treated in the same manner. Recurrent meatal warts should make the clinician suspect intraurethral warts and may be confirmed by urethroscopy. Intraurethral 5% 5-fluorouracil or thiotepa can be used but data are unavailable for prognosis (avoid podophyllin).

Pediculosis Pubis (Pubic Lice)

Lindane 1% lotion or cream is applied to involved areas and should be washed after 8 hours. Lindane 1% shampoo is indicated for hair involvement and should be applied for 4 to 5 minutes with thorough washing postadministration. Do not use in pregnant or lactating women. Retreatment is indicated after 7 days if lice or eggs are observed. Associated treatment is essential and includes washing and drying of clothing and bed linen. Sexual contacts should be treated as above.

SEXUALLY ABUSED CHILDREN AND RAPE VICTIMS

Any sexually transmitted infection (organism isolation or serology) out of the neonatal period should be considered as evidence of sexual abuse until proven otherwise. Sexual abuse is handled by an experienced physician or an experienced team of professionals. The actual risk of acquiring an STD in a sexual abuse case is less than in a rape victim, which is felt to be low.

TABLE 15-12. EVALUATION OF SEXUALLY ABUSED CHILDREN

Neisseria gonorrhea cultures from any potentially infected site

Chlamydia trachomatis cultures from any potentially infected site

Examination of vaginal specimens for trichomonas

Bimanual pelvic examination in postmenarchal sexually active women

Serologic test for syphilis and repeat in 2 mo

Serum sample frozen and saved for future testing

Examination of the assailant for evidence of STD, if available

Treatment is indicated when disease is present or laboratory test results are positive; prophylactic treatment is not recommended unless there is evidence that the assailant is infected

The Immune Compromised Host

NEONATES

The largest group of patients with immune deficiency are newborn infants. A number of defects have been documented during this age period that predispose these otherwise healthy neonates to life-threatening illness. It is not clear as to which defects might be relatively more important and which may be related to specific disease processes. The absence of immunoglobulin M is considered one of the more important deficiencies and one that at least partially accounts for propensity to gram-negative bacterial meningitis and sepsis (see Chap. 2).

**TABLE 16-1. MATURATIONAL DEFECTS OF
IMMUNITY IN NEONATES**

Humoral	Phagocytosis
IgM	Inflammatory response
IgA	Intracellular killing of
Complement levels	bacteria
Specific antibody production	Viral killing by monocytes
	PMN and monocyte
Cell-mediated	chemotaxis
Skin test responses	Random migration of
Suppressor cell activity	phagocytes
(increased)	PMN deformability
	Generation of serum
	chemotactic factors

The newborn is particularly vulnerable to treatment modalities
that may further depress his or her immune function. Splenectomy is associated with a much higher long-term morbidity in the
neonate as compared to older children and adults, and steroid
therapy, similarly, is fraught with more complications in this age
group. The trauma of surgery and thermal burns both suppress
immune function in patients of all ages, but in neonates they may
have a more potent influence on immune capabilities with resulting fatal infection.

Most of the basic principles that apply to the management of
immune compromised patients are relevant to neonates. Maximum doses of bactericidal antibiotics should be given with duration of therapy often being longer than for similar disease in
infants and children.

IATROGENIC FACTORS

Secondary immune deficiency is often iatrogenically introduced.
Chemotherapeutic regimens for cancer patients directed at inhib-
iting tumor replication are, at the same time, toxic to all elements
in the bone marrow, including immunologically competent
WBCs. In addition, patients with a variety of diseases are kept

alive for a longer period of time using extraordinary supportive measures that offer a much greater chance for eventual colonization with multiresistant or unusual microorganisms and eventual overt infectious disease. The infectious agents which cause such disease are often opportunistic organisms.

With each medical intervention in these fragile patients, the physician must calculate risk factors and anticipate complications. Some common complications involve local factors related to diagnostic or therapeutic procedures and to the placement of indwelling catheters, cannulae, or other foreign bodies. This sets the stage for colonization with opportunistic pathogens, which may then account for significant morbidity and mortality.

TABLE 16-2. IATROGENICALLY INDUCED PREDISPOSITION TO INFECTION

Local factors—mucosal and skin lesions
   Drugs (e.g., cyclophosphamide)
   Procedures (IV, cutdown, bone marrow, biopsy)
   Surgical wounds
Urinary catheters
Intravascular devices (IV, intraarterial, CVP, Swan-Ganz, etc.)
Respiratory support (ventilator, IPPB, etc.)
Transfusion transmitted disease
Splenectomy
Hospital-acquired resistant bacteria (lack of handwashing)

Most patients with diseases which result in secondary immunodeficiency receive blood or blood products during the course of their therapy. The transmission of infectious diseases to these patients represents a significant risk, particularly if multiple transfusions are given. It should be noted that many of these agents are not routinely screened in potential blood donors. Hepatitis represents the one best understood and most carefully monitored disease, whereas recent literature incriminates cytomegalovirus as an agent that is increasingly likely to cause severe illness. Blood donors are often asymptomatic for infectious agents at the time of phlebotomy. In the compromised host, additional care should be taken in screening donors and in providing follow-up medical examination of donors as a routine aspect of the recipient's care. Additional problems with transfusion therapy are pulmonary edema from volume overload, hemolytic reactions, and other incompletely understood febrile reactions.

TABLE 16–3. INFECTIONS TRANSMITTED BY BLOOD TRANSFUSIONS

Bacterial	Other
Bacterial sepsis	Toxoplasmosis
Endotoxemia	Syphilis
Brucellosis	Malaria
Salmonella	Leptospirosis
Viral	Filariasis
HAV	Trypanosomiasis
HBV	
Hepatitis non-A, non-B	
CMV	
Infectious mononucleosis	
Measles	
Rubella	
Colorado tick fever	
AIDS	

PRIMARY IMMUNE DEFICIENCY

It is difficult to determine the incidence of primary immune deficiency syndromes because many of the more severe forms may result in early infant death before diagnosis is made. In one British study, it was estimated that one of every 50 deaths in children was a result of immune dysfunction. Realistically, the more severe defects are only occasionally encountered by primary care physicians.

The more common deficiencies, such as transient hypogammaglobulinemia of infancy and selective IgA deficiency, are familiar to most clinicians. Most present during infancy or early childhood with the most notable exceptions being common variable hypogammaglobulinemia, cyclic neutropenia, and complement deficiencies which may not become clinically apparent until later in life. The deficiencies of the latter components of complement (C5-8) are not seen until adolescence or early adulthood with the presentation of recurrent meningococcal and gonococcal disease.

TABLE 16–4. PRIMARY IMMUNE DEFICIENCY SYNDROMES IN ORDER OF THEIR FREQUENCY

	Usual Age at Diagnosis	Gender
Transient hypogammaglobulinemia of infancy	6–12 mo	Both
Selective IgA deficiency	4–16 yr	Both
Common variable hypogammaglobulinemia	All ages	Both
Chronic mucocutaneous candidiasis	1–2 yr	Both
Cyclic neutropenia	All ages	Both
X-linked hypogammaglobulinemia (Bruton's)	6–12 mo	Male
Ataxia telangiectasia	3–5 yr	Both
Chronic granulomatous disease	2 yr	Male
SCID	9 mo	Both
Wiskott-Aldrich syndrome	1–2 yr	Male
Thymic hypoplasia (DiGeorge syndrome)	3 mo	Both
Complement deficiencies	All ages	Both

The approach to therapy varies according to specific defects demonstrated. The most difficult deficiencies to manage are those with T lymphocyte or combined T- and B-lymphocyte abnormality where either thymus or bone marrow transplantation represents definitive therapy. Selective B-lymphocyte deficiencies with hypogammaglobulinemia are treated with immunoglobulin replacement and this is best managed by the primary care physician. Both IM and IV preparations of human immune serum globulin are available for therapy. These should be used only for patients with documented hypogammaglobulinemia accompanied by recurrent clinical infection or with demonstrated inability to produce specific antibody following antigenic challenge (e.g., tetanus). The "physiologic" hypogammaglobulinemia apparent at 3 to 6 months of age does not require supplemental gammaglobulin and must be distinguished from transient hypogammaglobulinemia of infancy. The latter deficiency represents a delay of normal antibody synthesis after maternal IgG is no longer at protective levels; these infants may require immunoglobulin supplementation until approximately 18 months of age.

TABLE 16–5. THERAPEUTIC APPROACHES TO IMMUNE DEFICIENCY SYNDROMES

Syndrome	Therapy
T-cell deficiency	
DiGeorge syndrome (thymic aplasia	Thymus transplantation
Nezelof's syndrome (thymic hypoplasia)	Thymosin
Wiskott-Aldrich syndrome	Bone marrow transplantation
	Transfer factor
Ataxia telangiectasia	Fresh plasma
	Antibiotics
Chronic mucocutaneous candidiasis	Transfer factor
	Ketoconazole
B-cell deficiency	
Hypogammaglobulinemia	Immunoglobulin
Selective IgA deficiency	Antibiotics
Complement deficiencies	Antibiotics
	Fresh plasma
T- and B-cell deficiency	
Severe combined immune deficiency	Bone marrow transplantation
Histiocytosis X	Crude thymus extract
	Plasmapheresis

TABLE 16-5. (continued)

Syndrome	Therapy
Phagocytosis	
Chronic granulomatous disease	Antibiotics
	Bone marrow transplantation
Neutropenia	Antibiotics
	Granulocyte transfusions

TABLE 16-6. IMMUNOGLOBULIN REPLACEMENT FOR HYPOGAMMAGLOBULINEMIA

IgG Level	Patient Condition	Immunoglobulin Therapy
<250 mg/dl	Asymptomatic	0.66 ml/kg IM or 200 mg/kg IV q3-4wk
250-500 mg/dl	Asymptomatic	None
250-500 mg/dl	Infected	0.66 ml/kg IM or 200 mg/kg IV
>500 mg/dl	Infected	None

Defects in neutrophil function are characteristically followed closely with antibiotics offered for acute infectious episodes. Close communication must be maintained between patient and physician, which becomes the most important aspect of management.

SECONDARY IMMUNE DEFICIENCY

Suppression of immunologic function with resulting increased susceptibility to infection may occur as a result of a number of primary diseases. This circumstance is more common in adults than in children because of the higher incidence of malignancy and greater use of immunosuppressive chemotherapy for a variety of diseases.

Greater than 2% of all hospitalized children demonstrate secondary immune deficiency with the most common manifestation being hypogammaglobulinemia. Recognition and treatment of immunodeficiency has therefore become a very important aspect of hospital practice. Secondary deficiency is actually much more common than primary immunologic disorders, even in infants and children, and is usually managed by primary care physicians with the support of consultation.

TABLE 16-7. MOST COMMON CAUSES OF SECONDARY IMMUNODEFICIENCY IN CHILDREN

Sickle cell disease	Poor nutrition
Leukemia	Other malignancies
Nephrotic syndrome	Autoimmune disease
Down's syndrome	Immunosuppressive chemotherapy
Splenectomy	

Recognition of associations between specific infectious processes and primary disease offers important guidance to diagnosis and treatment. All of these should be well-understood by the physician caring for pediatric patients.

TABLE 16-8. UNUSUAL PATHOGENS AND DISEASE ENTITIES ASSOCIATED WITH SECONDARY IMMUNE DEFICIENCY

Leukemia	Disseminated chickenpox
	Pneumocystic carinii pneumonia
	Herpes simplex
	Candida sepsis
	Ecthyma gangrenosum *(Pseudomonas, Aeromonas)*
	Aspergillus pneumonia
Sickle cell disease	Pneumococcal meningitis, bacteremia and pneumonia
	Salmonella osteomyelitis

TABLE 16-8. (continued)

Nephrotic syndrome	Pneumococcal peritonitis
	Disseminated chickenpox
Down's syndrome	Pneumococcal pneumonia
	Hepatitis
Splenectomy	Pneumococcal sepsis
Diabetes	Malignant external otitis (*Pseudomonas*)
	Phycomycosis (mucormycosis)
	Listeriosis

Neutropenia

The congenital neutropenias may present either in childhood or during the adult years. These syndromes are secondary to inadequate production of granulocytes and, although a large spectrum of clinical consequences have been described, most patients do not appreciate a significantly increased propensity to infection. These syndromes include benign neutropenia with variants thereof, cyclic neutropenia, and what is termed infantile genetic agranulocytosis. Inadequate production of neutrophil precursors may also be the consequence of nutritional deficiencies, including vitamin B_{12} and folate, and secondary to infectious processes such as typhoid fever, infectious mononucleosis, and viral hepatitis. More common in adults are neutropenic states secondary to cytotoxic drugs used in therapy of cancer, autoimmune disease, and excessive destruction of granulocytes, either as inherited disorders, hypersplenism, or as a result of artificial heart valves or hemodialysis.

More recently described is an autoimmune process where antibodies, directed at neutrophils, produce profound neutropenia. These autoantibodies are often seen in conjunction with autoimmune states such as lupus erythematosus and Felty's syndrome. Infectious diseases are difficult to manage and account for the observed high mortality. Granulocyte transfusions are of no benefit because antineutrophil antibodies destroy donor cells. The clinical approach is careful monitoring for infectious episodes and early institution of antimicrobial therapy. Once acute infection is documented, these patients must be treated for much longer periods of time because it is so difficult to eradicate bacteria without the help of the host's granulocyte killing capacity.

Normal neutrophil counts are generally in the range of 2000 to 5000/mm^3 with variations accounted for by age, gender, and race. Although neutropenia is defined as an absolute neutrophil count less than 1500/mm^3, increased infection is not observed until a neutrophil count falls below 1000/mm^3. The absolute neutrophil count is an important objective parameter for making clinical decisions for patients with fever in the face of neutropenia. It has become a fairly standard protocol to offer antibiotics pending results of culture to these febrile patients who have a neutrophil count less than 500/mm^3.

During periods of anticipated transient neutropenia, such as during induction therapy for cancer, patients may benefit from granulocyte transfusions. This is simply not practical unless the period of neutropenia is 6 weeks or less but, under these defined conditions, benefits from such transfusions have been demonstrated.

TABLE 16–9. SUSCEPTIBILITY STAGING FOR NEUTROPENIA

Absolute Neutrophil Count	Predisposition to Bacterial Infection
> 1000/mm^3	Little
500-1000/mm^3	Mild
< 500/mm^3	Moderate (50%)
< 100/mm^3	Severe (100%)

Neutropenia and Fever

The most common clinical circumstance where the physician must make decisions for the immune compromised host is fever in the neutropenic patient. For pediatrics, this individual is most likely a child with leukemia who is neutropenic secondary to chemotherapy administered during treatment of the oncologic process. These patients are not only neutropenic, but their remaining granulocytes function poorly in mechanisms of phagocytosis and bacterial killing, unlike other neutropenic states, e.g., congenital neutropenia where remaining neutrophils function normally. This accounts for the increased susceptibility of neutropenic cancer patients over those with neutropenia of other etiology.

The best indicator of susceptibility to systemic bacterial disease is the absolute granulocyte count as previously outlined in Table 16-9. A count of less than $500/mm^3$ in a febrile patient dictates empiric antimicrobial therapy. If therapy is not instituted and blood cultures are obtained daily for 5 days, 50 to 80% will eventually demonstrate bacteremia. If antibiotics are not started until a positive culture is obtained, mortality under these circumstances is more than 80%.

TABLE 16-10. DOCUMENTED ETIOLOGY OF INFECTION IN CHILDHOOD LEUKEMIA

Bacteria	75%	Common bacterial pathogens	(75%)
Viral	20%	*Escherichia coli*	25%
VZV	7%	*Pseudomonas aeruginosa*	15%
HSV	5%	*Klebsiella-Enterobacter*	10%
CMV	5%	*Staphylococcus aureus*	10%
Fungal	5%	Others	15%
Candida albicans	4%		

Diagnostic evaluation should include cultures of blood, urine, stool, throat, and any suspicious focus, chest x-rays and lumbar puncture if CNS infection cannot be ruled out clinically. Baseline liver enzymes, renal function studies, and serum electrolytes should also be obtained prior to beginning antimicrobial therapy.

Selection of antibiotics must obviously provide coverage for the most likely pathogens yet particularly be directed at the most difficult-to-treat organisms. In most settings, *Pseudomonas aeruginosa* represents the most resistant organism.

TABLE 16-11. INITIAL EMPIRIC THERAPY FOR THE NEUTROPENIC FEBRILE PATIENT

Broad Spectrum Penicillin	*OR* Cephalosporin	*PLUS* Aminoglycoside
Carbenicillin	Ceftazidime	Gentamicin
Ticarcillin	Cephalothin	Tobramycin
Mezlocillin	Cefazolin	Amikacin
Piperacillin	Cefotaxime	Netilmicin
	Ceftriaxone	
	Moxalactam	

Aminoglycoside serum levels should be monitored in all patients to assure optimal but nontoxic levels of this antibiotic.

There is presently no clinical evidence that one particular combination from the list in Table 16-11 is more efficacious than another.

The last general comment is that the duration of recommended therapy is different from that for routine infections; treatment courses are dependent on the duration of the granulocytopenia. If a patient has return of peripheral neutrophils after only a few days of therapy, then antibiotics could be discontinued when the neutrophil count is adequate. On the other hand, if the granulocytopenia persists, discontinuing antibiotics can be dangerous for the patient, even after what would normally be considered adequate therapy.

The approach to therapy in the persistently neutropenic patient with continued fever, signs of infection, but negative cultures is a difficult one. Most authorities recommend an empiric change in antibiotics after 5 to 7 days with the addition of amphotericin B if the condition does not improve in 10 to 14 days.

TABLE 16-12. NEUTROPENIC PATIENTS WITH CONTINUED FEVER AND NEGATIVE CULTURES

Treatment Day	Therapy
0	Initial therapy (Table 16–11)
5–7	Another combination (Table 16–11)
	OR
	Clindamycin *PLUS*
	chloramphenicol
	OR
	TMP-SMX
10–14	Add amphotericin B

Candida Sepsis

Recovery of *Candida* sp. from the blood in immunosuppressed patients has become commonplace, usually the result of two predisposing factors: long-term, broad spectrum antibiotics and the presence of intravascular access lines. In almost all cases, catheters or other offending "foreign bodies" must be removed to eradicate this fungus. Consideration must also be given to limiting the number or spectrum of antimicrobial agents. Amphotericin B in relatively low doses and short duration is usually effective in the treatment of this infection. In the immunologically normal host with candidemia, removal of the intravascular line is often the only step necessary.

TABLE 16-13. MANAGEMENT OF CANDIDA SEPSIS

Predisposing factors
    Broad spectrum antibiotics
    Intravascular lines, urinary catheters or other foreign bodies
    GI colonization
    Surgery
Treatment
    Remove foreign body
    Adjust antimicrobial therapy
    Oral nystatin or ketoconazole for thrush or colonization
    Amphotericin B 0.5 mg/kg/day div qd × 14 days

PROPHYLAXIS

Some infections in well-defined immunosuppressed hosts are frequent enough to warrant prophylactic therapy. Circumstances for prophylaxis in the immunologically normal host are reviewed in Chapter 3.

TABLE 16–14. PROPHYLAXIS FOR THE IMMUNE COMPROMISED HOST

Underlying Disease	Infectious Agent	Prophylactic Regimen
Leukemia Primary immune deficiency SCID DiGeorge syndrome Nezelof's syndrome	*Pneumocystis carinii*	TMP-SMX 4 mg TMP/20 mg SMX/kg/day PO div q12h
Asplenia Splenectomy Sickle cell disease Complement deficiencies C_2, C_3, C_{3b} inhibitor, C_5	*S. pneumoniae*	Benzathine penicillin G 1.2 million U IM q3wk (>60 lb); 600,000 U (<60 lb) *OR* Penicillin V 250 mg PO bid (>60 lb) 125 mg (<60 lb)
Chronic granulomatous disease	*Staphylococcus aureus*	TMP-SMX 4 mg TMP/20 mg SMX kg/day PO div q12h

CUTANEOUS ANERGY

Transient defects in cell-mediated immunity are commonly encountered during the course of acute or chronic illnesses. For a variable period of time, patients may fail to demonstrate positive delayed hypersensitivity to intradermal skin testing. This presents an enigma to the clinician if he or she is using a skin test to diagnose the patient's primary illness. It is then impossible to differentiate whether a negative skin test represents cutaneous anergy or rules out a particular disease such as tuberculosis. For example, a patient with leukemia who develops a pulmonary infiltrate compatible with tuberculosis should have evaluation of cutaneous anergy along with the tuberculin skin test. There are many ways that this can be accomplished. A battery of skin tests might be applied along with tuberculin. A positive skin test to tetanus, candida, mumps, or SKSD, along with a negative tuberculin skin test would reassure the physician that this patient can respond to specific antigen and then interpret the negative tuberculin skin test as evidence against pulmonary tuberculosis. Because the PHA skin test is probably the most sensitive for evaluating anergy, a more rapid resolution of the question would be achieved with this mitogen in the initial skin test battery. Placing other skin tests first would mean a delay of 2 days prior to reading these tests if the PHA skin test is then applied as a second step in the diagnostic workup.

TABLE 16-15. CAUSES OF CUTANEOUS ANERGY

Primary immune deficiency	Infectious diseases
Secondary immune deficiency	Bacterial
Malignancy	Viral
Immunosuppressive	Fungal
therapy	Rickettsial
Autoimmune disease	Chronic diseases
Surgery (recent)	Sarcoidosis
Trauma	Rheumatoid
Burns	Renal diseases
Poor nutritional status	Alcoholism
Advanced age	Cirrhosis
Acute disease processes	Diabetes

It is always better to have monitored patients with diseases known to be associated with cutaneous anergy so that, if a clinical circumstance arises requiring skin testing, no time is lost. In addition, documentation of cutaneous anergy would then alert the

physician that this patient is highly predisposed to infectious processes. It should be emphasized that the degree of cellular immune suppression is critical in determining the patient's
predisposition to secondary infectious processes. This can be
roughly quantitated by performing in vitro antigen and mitogen
stimulation in addition to skin testing of patients. Its importance
for clinical management is to direct early and aggressive use of
antifungal or antituberculous medication for the severely immunosuppressed individual, often prior to receiving final culture results. Using this staging system, patients can be categorized into
those who have mild suppression of cellular immunity as manifested only by negative skin tests to specific antigens as contrasted
to the severely immune suppressed individuals who have negative
skin test responses to antigens, PHA, negative in vitro antigen induced lymphocyte stimulation responses, and a PHA mitogen
lymphocyte stimulation response less than 10% of control. The
latter patients are at extremely high risk to infection with opportunistic pathogens, particularly fungi and herpes group viruses.

TABLE 16-16. WORKUP OF CUTANEOUS ANERGY AND SUSCEPTIBILITY STAGING OF PATIENTS

	Degree of Immune Suppression if Tests Negative

1. Skin testing
  a. Tetanus toxoid 1:1
  b. Dermatophytin O (*Candida*) 1:10
  c. SK/SD 40U/10U
	1+

2. Skin testing with PHA—20 μg dose	2+
3. In vitro antigen (e.g., *Candida*) induced lymphocyte stimulation	3+
4. In vitro mitogen (e.g., PHA) induced lymphocyte stimulation 10-50% of control	4+
5. In vitro mitogen (e.g., PHA) induced lymphocyte stimulation 10% of control	5+

RECURRENT STAPHYLOCOCCAL INFECTION: TREATMENT WITH BACTERIAL INTERFERENCE

Intact skin and mucous membranes with their normal bacterial microflora constitute the host's primary defense against invasion by microbial agents. Any alteration of colonizing bacteria may result in covert or overt infectious processes. Furuncles and subcutaneous abscesses result from a breakdown in this basic immune mechanism and account for as many as one in every 50 visits to hospital emergency facilities. Moreover, skin infections tend to be recurrent in many patients and often spread to other family members. Medical intervention is most appropriately directed toward eradication of the offending organism and for recurrent infections, toward strengthening the patient's resistance to infection. In this instance, resistance is provided by the individual's colonizing microflora.

Previous studies have demonstrated that purposeful colonization with the penicillin sensitive 502A strain of *Staphylococcus aureus* interferes with subsequent colonization by more virulent strains of *S. aureus* in neonates and adults. Protection against recurrent intrafamilial furunculosis by nasal inoculation of *Staphylococcus* 502A has also been reported. Essentially, the mechanism is, in part, restoration of the host's primary immune barrier against infection, i.e., noninvasive bacterial microflora.

Table 16-17 outlines a simple protocol for treating patients with recurrent cutaneous abscesses. A single nasal inoculum of *S. aureus* 502A following therapy directed at reducing colonization with more virulent *S. aureus* organisms will subsequently prevent reinfection. This approach has been referred to previously as "artificial colonization" or "bacterial interference." This method is quite practical and could be employed in most outpatient facilities. The only equipment requirements are a standard freezer compartment and a small 37C incubator. Aliquots of *S. aureus* 502A in trypticase soy broth or sheep red cells may be readily prepared in a local microbiologic laboratory and sent to the clinician for storage and subsequent use.

TABLE 16–17. PROTOCOL FOR TREATING RECURRENT CUTANEOUS ABSCESSES

Patient
    Incision and drainage of active lesions
    Erythromycin PO × 7–14 days

Patient and family members
    bid hexachlorophene showers × 7–14 days
    bid nasal topical bacitracin × 7–14 days
    2 days off nasal bacitracin
    Nasal colonization with *S. aureus* 502A

The initial treatment of cutaneous abscesses often involves incision and drainage, with the necessity for antibiotics given for systemic effect remaining debatable; the aerobe most prevalent in recovery from cutaneous abscesses is *S. aureus*. A recent report demonstrated that there was no apparent diagnostic benefit achieved by employing routine gram stains or cultures of such infections nor therapeutic efficacy following antimicrobial therapy. The combination of these diagnostic and therapeutic procedures is quite expensive and the nature of cutaneous abscesses would require repeated treatment. Bacterial interference is thus more effective, less expensive, and quite applicable for primary care physicians.

Similar GI therapeutic colonization with selected benign microflora is currently being employed for patients who have undergone bone marrow transplantation or those recovering from aggressive immunosuppressive chemotherapy. This provides colonizing bacteria that are nonvirulent and less likely to cause systemic infection in the compromised host.

Infection Control

Infections in Pediatric Hospital Personnel
Mechanisms of Disease Transmission
Control Measures
Isolation Policies

INFECTIONS IN PEDIATRIC HOSPITAL PERSONNEL

The hospital provides an environment of unique microorganisms (antibiotic-resistant) and susceptible individuals (immunosuppressed). In such a setting, hospital personnel are exposed to multiple agents and patients, and may serve as vectors for disease transmission.

TABLE 17-1. INFECTIONS FOR WHICH PEDIATRIC PERSONNEL ARE AT SPECIAL RISK

Bacteria	Viruses
Staphylococcus	Hepatitis A and B
Pertussis	Adenovirus
Streptococcus	Rubella
Meningococcus	HSV
Mycobacteria	CMV
	Rotavirus

MECHANISMS OF DISEASE TRANSMISSION

Hospital infections are transmitted by airborne dissemination, exposure to a contaminated common vehicle, and person-to-person contact. Because the pediatric patient is usually an ineffective aerosolizer, hands of hospital personnel become the most important vehicles for carrying microorganisms from one patient to another.

CONTROL MEASURES

Prevention of infections acquired during hospitalization is a goal of all physicians. A firm understanding of the mechanisms of disease transmission is foremost in infection control.

TABLE 17–2. INFECTION CONTROL MEASURES TO PREVENT HOSPITAL-ACQUIRED INFECTIONS

Recognition of infectious process
Appropriate treatment of infection
Proper handling of patient and body secretions
Isolation
Handwashing

ISOLATION POLICIES

Isolation policies must be modified to meet the needs of individual hospitals. For the purposes of this book, representative diseases as outlined in the Centers for Disease Control manual *Guidelines for Prevention and Control of Nosocomial Infections* have been selected to illustrate disease-specific isolation techniques.

TABLE 17-3. DISEASE-SPECIFIC ISOLATION PRECAUTIONS

Disease	Precautions Indicated					Infective Material	Apply Precautions (How Long?)
	Private Room?	Masks?	Gowns?	Gloves?			
Abscess, etiology unknown							
Draining, major	Yes	No	Yes, if soiling is likely	Yes, for touching infective material		Pus	Duration of illness
Comments: Major—no dressing or dressing does not adequately contain the pus							
Draining, minor or limited	No	No	Yes, if soiling is likely	Yes, for touching infective material		Pus	Duration of illness
Comments: Minor or limited—dressing covers and adequately contains the pus, or infected area is small, such as a stitch abscess							
Bronchiolitis, etiology unknown in infants and young children	Yes	No	Yes, if soiling is likely	No		Respiratory secretions	Duration of illness
Comments: Various etiologic agents, such as respiratory syncytial virus, parainfluenza viruses, adenoviruses, and influenza viruses, have been associated with this syndrome (Committee on Infectious Diseases, American Academy of Pediatrics, 1982, Red Book); therefore, precautions to prevent their spread are generally indicated							

(continued)

345

TABLE 17-3. (continued)

| Disease | Precautions Indicated | | | | | Infective Material | Apply Precautions (How Long?) |
	Private Room?	Masks?	Gowns?	Gloves?			
Bronchitis, infective etiology unknown							
Infants and young children	Yes	No	Yes, if soiling is likely	No		Respiratory secretions	Duration of illness
Other	No	No	No	No			
Chickenpox (Varicella)	Yes	Yes	Yes	Yes		Respiratory secretions and lesion secretions	Until all lesions are crusted

Comments: Persons who are not susceptible do not need to wear a mask. Susceptible persons should, if possible, stay out of room. Special ventilation for the room, if available, may be advantageous, especially for outbreak control. Neonates born to mothers with active varicella should be placed on isolation precautions at birth. Exposed susceptible patients should be placed on isolation precautions beginning 10 days after exposure and continuing until 21 days after last exposure. See CDC Guideline for Infection Control in Hospital Personnel for recommendations for exposed susceptible personnel

TABLE 17-3. (continued)

					Respiratory secretions	Duration of illness
Common cold Infants and young children	Yes	No	Yes, if soiling is likely	No	Respiratory secretions	Duration of illness

Comments: Although rhinoviruses are most frequently associated with the common cold and are mild in adults, severe infections may occur in infants and young children. Other etiologic agents, such as respiratory syncytial viruses, may also cause this syndrome (Committee on Infectious Diseases, American Academy of Pediatrics, 1982, Red Book); therefore, precautions to prevent their spread are generally indicated

					Respiratory secretions	Duration of illness
Croup	Yes	No	Yes, if soiling is likely	No	Respiratory secretions	Duration of illness

Comments: Because viral agents, such as parainfluenza and influenza A virus, have been associated with this syndrome (Committee on Infectious Diseases, American Academy of Pediatrics, 1982, Red Book), precautions to prevent their spread are generally indicated

(continued)

TABLE 17-3. (continued)

Disease	Precautions Indicated					Infective Material	Apply Precautions (How Long?)
	Private Room?	Masks?	Gowns?	Gloves?			
CMV infection neonatal or immunosuppressed	No	No	No	No		Urine and respiratory secretions may be	
Comments: Pregnant personnel may need special counseling (see CDC Guideline for Infection Control in Hospital Personnel)							
Epiglottitis, due to Haemophilus influenzae	Yes	Yes, for those close to patient	No	No		Respiratory secretions	For 24 hr after start of effective therapy
Gastroenteritis Campylobacter sp.	Yes, if patient hygiene is poor	No	Yes, if soiling is likely	Yes, for touching infective material		Feces	Duration of illness
Clostridium difficile	Yes, if patient hygiene is poor	No	Yes, if soiling is likely	Yes, for touching infective material		Feces	Duration of illness

Organism						
Escherichia coli (enteropathogenic, enterotoxic or enteroinvasive)	Yes, if patient hygiene is poor	No	Yes, if soiling is likely	Yes, for touching infective material	Feces	Duration of illness
Giardia lamblia	Yes, if patient hygiene is poor	No	Yes, if soiling is likely	Yes, for touching infective material	Feces	Duration of illness
Rotavirus	Yes, if patient hygiene is poor	No	Yes, if soiling is likely	Yes, for touching infective material	Feces	Duration of illness or 7 days after onset, whichever is less
Salmonella sp.	Yes, if patient hygiene is poor	No	Yes, if soiling is likely	Yes, for touching infective material	Feces	Duration of illness

(continued)

TABLE 17-3. (continued)

	Precautions Indicated						
Disease	Private Room?	Masks?	Gowns?	Gloves?	Infective Material	Apply Precautions (How Long?)	
Shigella sp.	Yes, if patient hygiene is poor	No	Yes, if soiling is likely	Yes, for touching infective material	Feces	Until 3 consecutive cultures of feces taken after ending antimicrobial therapy are negative for infecting strain	
Unknown etiology	Yes, if patient hygiene is poor	No	Yes, if soiling is likely	Yes, for touching infective material	Feces	Duration of illness	
Vibrio parahaemolyticus	Yes, if patient hygiene is poor	No	Yes, if soiling is likely	Yes, for touching infective material	Feces	Duration of illness	
Viral	Yes, if patient hygiene is poor	No	Yes, if soiling is likely	Yes, for touching infective material	Feces	Duration of illness	

						Duration of illness
Yersinia enterocolitica	Yes, if patient hygiene is poor	No	Yes, if soiling is likely	Yes, for touching infective material	Feces	
Meningitis						
Aseptic (nonbacterial or viral meningitis) (also see specific etiologies)	Yes, if patient hygiene is poor	No	Yes, if soiling is likely	Yes, for touching infective material	Feces	For 7 days after onset
Comments: Enteroviruses are the most common cause of aseptic meningitis						
Bacterial, gram-negative enteric in neonates	No	No	No	No	Feces	

Comments: During a nursery outbreak, cohort ill and colonized infants, and use gowns if soiling likely and gloves when touching feces

(continued)

TABLE 17–3. (continued)

| Disease | Precautions Indicated | | | | Infective Material | Apply Precautions (How Long?) |
	Private Room?	Masks?	Gowns?	Gloves?		
Meningococcemia (meningococcal sepsis)	Yes	Yes, for those close to patient	No	No	Respiratory secretions	For 24 hr after start of effective therapy

Comments: See Chapter 3 for recommendations for prophylaxis after exposure

Pertussis ("whooping cough")	Yes	Yes, for those close to patient	No	No	Respiratory secretions	For 7 days after start of effective therapy

Comments: See Chapter 3 for recommendations for prophylaxis after exposure

18

Antimicrobial Therapy

EMPIRIC THERAPY

The initial selection of antimicrobial agents is usually made before definitive cultures and sensitivities are available. The physician must therefore first have an understanding of the pathogens that commonly cause the specific infectious process under consideration. Other chapters in this book discuss in greater detail anticipated etiologic agents. This must then be translated into initial empiric therapy. With the increasing number of newer agents presently entering the market, there are now many alternatives for this selection.

It is, of course, essential to first obtain all necessary gram stain and culture specimens before beginning treatment. In many cases, gram stains of body fluids (buffy coat, joint aspiration, CSF, urine, pleural effusion, etc.) will guide selection of antimicrobial agents.

TABLE 18-1. INITIAL EMPIRIC THERAPY FOR SERIOUS NEONATAL INFECTIONS (birth–3 mo)

Disease			Antibiotics
Sepsis or meningitis (Chap. 2)	Ampicillin	*PLUS*	Ceftriaxone, cefotaxime, moxalactam, or gentamicin
NEC (Chap. 3)	Clindamycin, chloramphenicol, or moxalactam	*PLUS*	Ampicillin, ticarcillin, or mezlocillin
		PLUS	Gentamicin or amikacin
Osteomyelitis (Chap. 9)	Methicillin and ceftriaxone		
Peritonitis (Chap. 14)	Ampicillin, gentamicin and clindamycin		
Pneumonia (Chap. 7)	Methicillin	*PLUS*	Ceftriaxone cefotaxime, moxalactam, or gentamicin
Septic arthritis (Chap. 9)	Methicillin	*PLUS*	Ceftriaxone
UTI (Chap. 10)	Gentamicin		

TABLE 18-2. INITIAL EMPIRIC THERAPY IN INFANTS AND CHILDREN (> 3 mo)

Disease		Antibiotics
Sepsis and meningitis (Chap. 1)		Ceftriaxone, cefotaxime, ceftizoxime (>6 mo of age), or moxalactam + penicillin
Cellulitis (Chap. 4)		
Facial, orbital, preseptal		Ceftriaxone, cefotaxime or moxalactam
Facial (following trauma)		Nafcillin
Trunk or extremities		Nafcillin
3 mo–5 yr add		Ceftriaxone, cefotaxime, or moxalactam
Osteomyelitis (Chap. 9)	Nafcillin *PLUS*	Ceftriaxone, cefotaxime, or moxalactam
Foot (following trauma)	Ticarcillin *PLUS*	Gentamicin *PLUS* nafcillin
Otitis media (Chap. 4)		Amoxicillin
Pneumonia (Chap. 7)		
< 5 yr		Amoxicillin
5–10 yr		Penicillin
> 10 yr		Erythromycin
Severe or with empyema	Nafcillin *PLUS*	Ceftriaxone, cefotaxime, cefuroxime, or moxalactam
Septic arthritis (Chap. 9)		
< 7 yr	Nafcillin *PLUS*	Ceftriaxone, cefotaxime, or moxalactam
> 7 yr		Nafcillin
Shunt (VP) infections (Chap. 13)	Vancomycin *PLUS*	Ceftriaxone, cefotaxime, or moxalactam

(continued)

TABLE 18-2. (continued)

Disease	Antibiotics
Sinusitis (Chap. 7)	Amoxicillin
UTI (Chap. 10)	
Cystitis	Amoxicillin or sulfisoxazole
Pyelonephritis	Gentamicin or TMP/SMX

ADVERSE REACTIONS

An appreciation of untoward side effects is as important as a knowledge of the therapeutic potential of antibiotics. Because many are of equal efficacy, selection is often determined on the basis of relative toxicity. Third generation cephalosporins (ceftriaxone, cefotaxime, and moxalactam) are desirable because they circumvent the potential toxicity of chloramphenicol and aminoglycosides when treating *H. influenzae* or gram-negative coliform infection, respectively. Likewise, nafcillin is preferred over methicillin beyond the neonatal age range because nephrotoxicity is less common. Methicillin, however, should be used in neonates because nafcillin serum and tissue levels are erratic in this age group. Tetracyclines should be avoided in children less than 8 years of age as this drug is deposited in teeth and bones.

There is a narrow margin between therapeutic and toxic levels of chloramphenicol and aminoglycosides. Therefore, monitoring of peak and trough levels is essential for individual dosage adjustment. For most other antibiotics, toxic levels far exceed usual therapeutic ranges.

TABLE 18-3. RELATIVE FREQUENCY OF ALLERGIC REACTIONS TO COMMONLY USED ANTIBIOTICS

Highest	Sulfonamides
	Penicillins
	Cephalosporins
	Aminoglycosides
	Chloramphenicol
Lowest	Erythromycin

**TABLE 18–4. IMPORTANT ADVERSE REACTIONS
ASSOCIATED WITH ANTIBIOTICS**

Antibiotic	Reaction
All antibiotics	Overgrowth of resistant bacteria and fungi (*Candida albicans*)
	Hypersensitivity skin rashes
	Serum sickness
	Anaphylaxis
	Bone marrow toxicity
	Nephrotoxicity
	Pseudomembranous colitis
	Drug fever
Penicillins	
Ampicillin	Diarrhea
Carbenicillin	Platelet dysfunction
	Hypernatremia, hypokalemia
Ticarcillin, piperacillin, mezlocillin	Platelet dysfunction
Cephalosporins	Nephrotoxicity
	Direct Coomb's reaction (probably of no clinical significance)
	Phlebitis and phlebothrombosis
Cefaclor	Serum sickness-like reaction
Cefamandole	Antabuse effect
Moxalactam	Antabuse effect
	Bleeding in adults
Aminoglycosides	Nephrotoxicity
	Ototoxicity
	Neuromuscular blockade
Chloramphenicol	Aplastic anemia
	Circulatory collapse ("gray syndrome")
	Hypoplastic marrow
Tetracycline	Decreased bone growth and staining of teeth in children less than 8 yr of age
	Abdominal pain
	Diarrhea
	Pseudotumor cerebri
	Angioedema
	Brown tongue

(*continued*)

TABLE 18-4. (continued)

Antibiotic	Reaction
Tetracycline (*cont.*)	Glossitis
	Anal pruritis
	Fanconi's syndrome
Minocycline	Vestibular toxicity
Erythromycin	Nausea
	Abdominal pain
	Cholestatic hepatitis
	Phlebitis
Sulfonamides	Stevens-Johnson syndrome
TMP/SMX	Hypersensitivity skin rashes
	Stevens-Johnson syndrome
Rifampin	GI distress
	Thrombocytopenia

HOST FACTORS RELATED TO ANTIBIOTIC SELECTION

Compromised Host
Selection of antibiotics for the compromised host, particularly the granulocytopenic patient, requires three major alterations in prescribing practices. First, two agents rather than one should be given and these should be chosen for their potential synergism against the presumed or identified pathogen (Table 18-5). Maximum doses should then be employed. Finally, where alternatives are available, bactericidal rather than bacteriostatic agents should be given (Table 18-6). This is necessary because bacteriostatic agents primarily inhibit bacterial growth while relying on host factors for complete killing of the organisms. Following therapy with these agents in the compromised host, relapse is frequent. Bactericidal agents are much more effective in totally eliminating pathogens in the absence of adequate mechanisms of host defense.

TABLE 18-5. ANTIBIOTIC SYNERGISM

Pathogen	Synergistic Combination		
Pseudomonas aeruginosa	Aminoglyco-side	*PLUS*	A broad spectrum penicillin (carbenicillin, ticarcillin or piperacillin)
Staphylococcus aureus	Gentamicin	*PLUS*	Nafcillin
Enterococci	Gentamicin	*PLUS*	Penicillin, nafcillin, or vancomycin
Viridans streptococci	Gentamicin	*PLUS*	Penicillin or vancomycin
Klebsiella pneumoniae	Aminoglyco-side	*PLUS*	Cephalosporin
Coliforms (*E. coli, Enterobacter, Proteus* and *Providencia*)	Gentamicin	*PLUS*	Ampicillin, carbenicillin or cephalosporins
Mycobacterium tuberculosis	Isoniazid	*PLUS*	Rifampin

TABLE 18-6. IN VITRO CLASSIFICATION OF ANTIBIOTICS

Bactericidal	Bacteriostatic
Aminoglycosides	Chloramphenicol
Cephalosporins	Clindamycin
Penicillins	Erythromycin
Vancomycin	Sulfonamides
	Tetracyclines

Renal Failure

In patients with abnormal renal function, dosages of many antibiotics must be altered, relative to the degree of renal impairment. In many circumstances an antibiotic can be chosen that is excreted by extrarenal mechanisms, thereby avoiding potential increased toxicity. If such a selection cannot be made, it becomes even more critical to monitor drug serum levels.

There are two basic approaches to dosage modification: (a) increasing the dosing interval or (b) decreasing the individual dose. For severe infections, particularly with bacteremia, many experts recommend the latter approach, which would best assure more frequent high serum levels of antibiotic. This approach, however, is more likely to result in higher trough levels, which may increase the risk of nephrotoxicity for aminoglycosides. For most other infections, it is more prudent to increase the dosing interval and obtain peak and trough levels to further guide therapy.

**TABLE 18-7. DOSAGE MODIFICATION IN
RENAL FAILURE[a]**

Modification	Antibiotic
None	Penicillins
	Nafcillin
	Cloxacillin
	Dicloxacillin
	Cephalosporins
	Cefoperazone
	Ceftriaxone
	Chloramphenicol
	Erythromycin
	Tetracyclines
	Doxycycline
	Minocycline
	Isoniazid
	Rifampin
Give usual dose q12h	Penicillins (other than above)
	Cephalosporins (other than cefoperazone and ceftriaxone)

TABLE 18-7. (continued)

Modification	Antibiotic
Major (monitor levels)	TMP/SMX Clindamycin Aminoglycosides Vancomycin

[a] Creatinine clearance 10 ml/min.

Hepatic Failure

For patients with severe hepatic disease, antibiotics that are metabolized by the liver or excreted through the biliary tract should be avoided. Adequate guidelines for dosage modification are simply not available. The only approach, which might assure safe administration, is frequent measurement of serum drug levels.

TABLE 18-8. ANTIBIOTICS CONTRAINDICATED IN HEPATIC FAILURE

Cefoperazone
Chloramphenicol
Clindamycin
Erythromycin
Isoniazid
Nitrofurantoin
Rifampin
Tetracyclines

Penicillin Allergy and Desensitization

In patients with documented allergic reactions to penicillins, one of this class of antibiotics may still have to be given for certain life-threatening infections. The most common clinical circumstance is streptococcal or staphylococcal endocarditis. For most other severe infections (meningitis, pneumonia, etc.) cephalosporins or chloramphenicol represent adequate alternatives.

Penicillin allergy skin testing may first be undertaken to confirm hypersensitivity in a patient with a questionable history. Such testing is time consuming and with currently available reagents, yields a 5% false-negative and 80% false-positive reaction rate. Limitations to this testing are primarily attributable to the absence of a reliable minor determinant mixture (MDM). Major determinant, benzylpenicilloyl-polylysine (PPL), can be obtained through commercial sources (Pre-pen, Kremers-Urban, Milwaukee, Wis.). Some studies have used a fresh solution of crystalline penicillin G as the source of MDM. If the antibiotic to be given is a derivative of penicillin, skin testing should include this derivative in addition to testing with PPL and penicillin G. With each product, scratch testing should be followed by intradermal injection of 0.01 to 0.02 ml. For scratch testing, a drop of the test solution is placed on the forearm and a 3- to 5-mm scratch made at this site with a 20-gauge needle. For penicillin G or penicillin derivative testing serial scratch tests followed by serial intradermal injections with solutions of 0.25 mg/ml, 2.5 mg/ml, and 25 mg/ml are recommended. Each test should be observed for 15 minutes before proceeding to the next. A positive reaction is a wheal greater than 5 mm. Normal saline and histamine (1 mg/ml) should be included as negative and positive controls.

When a penicillin must be given to an allergic patient, desensitization, beginning with oral administration should be accomplished and this can be done with penicillin G or any derivative. This should be undertaken in the hospital where careful monitoring and treatment for allergic reactions are available.

TABLE 18-9. PENICILLIN DESENSITIZATION

Time	Dose (mg)	Units	Route
0	0.05	100	PO
15 min	0.10	200	PO
30 min	0.25	400	PO

TABLE 18-9. (continued)

Time	Dose (mg)	Units	Route
45 min	0.5	800	PO
1 hr	1	1,600	PO
1 hr 15 min	2	3,200	PO
1 hr 30 min	4	6,400	PO
1 hr 45 min	8	12,500	PO
2 hr	15	25,000	PO
2 hr 15 min	30	50,000	PO
2 hr 30 min	60	100,000	PO
2 hr 45 min	125	200,000	PO
3 hr	250	400,000	PO
3 hr 15 min	125	200,000	SC
3 hr 30 min	250	400,000	SC
3 hr 45 min	500	800,000	SC
4 hr	625	1,000,000	IM
4 hr 15 min	Begin full dose IV		

DOSAGES OF ANTIBIOTICS

Neonates

There are actually very few antibiotics commonly used for the treatment of neonatal infection. Pharmacokinetics, however, change rapidly during the first weeks of life and differ between prematurely born and full-term neonates. Dosages and intervals of administration must therefore be adjusted frequently during the course of treatment and this requirement represents the most unique feature of therapy in the neonatal patient. Among the semisynthetic penicillinase-resistant penicillins, methicillin is preferred because pharmacokinetics are less erratic. Selection of an aminoglycoside in a particular institution is more predicated on resistance patterns of coliforms for that institution than on pharmacokinetic differences. It is always necessary to monitor peak and trough levels of aminoglycosides so laboratory capabilities may influence choices among these agents.

TABLE 18-10 DAILY DOSAGES OF IV ANTIBIOTICS FOR NEONATES WITH SERIOUS INFECTIONS

Antibiotic	Full-Term Neonate	Premature Neonate
Amikacin	< 7 days 15 mg/kg div q12h > 7 days 20 mg/kg div q8h	15 mg/kg div q12h
Ampicillin	< 7 days 100 mg/kg div q12h > 7 days 200 mg/kg div q8h	100 mg/kg div q12h
Carbenicillin	< 3 days > 2000 g 300 mg/kg div q6h > 3 days > 2000 g 400 mg/kg div q6h	< 7 days and < 2000 g 225 mg/kg div q8h > 7 days and > 2000 g 400 mg/kg div q6h
Cefotaxime	< 7 days 100 mg/kg div q12h > 7 days 150 mg/kg div q8h	100 mg/kg div q12h
Ceftazidime	< 7 days 100 mg/kg div q12h > 7 days 150 mg/kg div q8h	100 mg/kg div q12h
Ceftriaxone	100 mg/kg div q12h	75 mg/kg div q12h
Cephalothin	< 7 days 40 mg/kg div q12h > 7 days 60 mg/kg div q8h	40 mg/kg div q12h
Chloramphenicol	< 2 wk 25 mg/kg div q8h > 2 wk 50 mg/kg div q6h	25 mg/kg div q8h
Clindamycin	20 mg/kg div q8h	15 mg/kg div q8h
Gentamicin	< 7 days 5 mg/kg div q12h > 7 days 7.5 mg/kg div q8h	5 mg/kg div q12h 1000–1500 g 2.5 mg/kg q18h < 1000 g 2.5 mg/kg q24h
Kanamycin	> 2000 g ≤ 7 days 20 mg/kg div q12h	< 2000 g ≤ 3 days 10 mg/kg div q24h

TABLE 18–10 (continued)

Antibiotic	Full-Term Neonate	Premature Neonate
	> 2000 g ≥ 8 days 30 mg/kg div q8h	< 2000 g ≥ 4 days 20 mg/kg div q12h
Methicillin	< 10 days 200 mg/kg div q8h > 10 days 200 mg/kg div q6h	< 10 days < 2500 g 100 mg/kg div q8h > 10 days < 2500 g 100 mg/kg div q6h
Metronidazole	15 mg/kg loading dose 15 mg/kg div q12h	
Mezlocillin	≤ 7 days > 2000 g 150 mg/kg div q12h > 7 days > 2000 g 300 mg/kg div q6h	≤ 7 days < 2000 g 150 mg/kg div q12h > 7 days < 2000 g 225 mg/kg div q8h
Moxalactam	≤ 7 days 100 mg/kg div q12h > 7 days 150 mg/kg div q8h	100 mg/kg div q12h
Penicillin G	< 7 days 250,000 U/kg div q8h > 7 days 400,000 U/kg div q6h	250,000 U/kg div q12h

Penicillin G, benzathine (IM) 50,000 U/kg as single dose IM for asymptomatic congenital syphilis
Penicillin G, aqueous (IM) 50,000 U/kg IV div q12h for symptomatic congenital syphilis

Ticarcillin	≤ 7 days 225 mg/kg div q8h > 7 days 300 mg/kg div q6h	≤ 7 days 150 mg/kg div q12h > 7 days 225 mg/kg div q8h
Tobramycin	≤ 7 days 4 mg/kg div q12h > 7 days 6 mg/kg div q8h	4 mg/kg div q12h
Vancomycin	≤ 7 days 30 mg/kg div q12h > 7 days 45 mg/kg div q8h	30 mg/kg div q12h

TABLE 18-11. DOSAGES OF ORAL ANTIBIOTICS FOR NEONATES

Antibiotic (Trade Name)	Daily Dosage
Amoxicillin (numerous trade names)	20-40 mg/kg div q8h
Ampicillin (numerous trade names)	50-100 mg/kg div q8h
Cefaclor (Ceclor)	40 mg/kg div q8h
Cephalexin (Keflex)	50 mg/kg div q6h
Chloramphenicol (Chloromycetin)	< 14 days 25 mg/kg div q8h > 14 days 50 mg/kg div q6h
Cloxacillin (Tegopen)	> 2500 g 50-100 mg/kg div q6h < 2500 g 50 mg/kg div q8h
Dicloxacillin (Dycill, Dynapen, Pathocil)	> 2500 g 50-100 mg/kg div q6h < 2500 g 50 mg/kg div q8h
Erythromycin (numerous trade names)	< 7 days 20 mg/kg div q12h > 7 days 20-40 mg/kg div q8h
Oxacillin (Bactocill, Prostaphlin)	> 2500 g 50-100 mg/kg div q6h < 2500 g 50 mg/kg div q8h
Penicillin V (numerous trade names)	50,000 U/kg div q8h

Infants and Children

After 28 days of age, pharmacokinetic patterns are quite constant although different from the adult who has a relatively smaller volume of distribution. This simply means that relatively higher amounts of antibiotics must be given to children to achieve the same serum concentrations. Dosages can be calculated according to weight for most children, exceptions being those with excessive obesity or malnutrition (cystic fibrosis and cancer patients). In these cases, dosages should be calculated by body surface area (see Table 18-15). For children over 12 years or weighing more than 40 kg, maximum dosage limitations should be reviewed (see Table 18-14).

Monitoring of drug levels for aminoglycosides and chloramphenicol should be accomplished for patients who will be kept on these antimicrobial agents for more than 48 hours (when initial culture information is available). Other antibiotic concentrations may be indirectly measured by performing serum bactericidal assays with the recovered pathogen. These assays should be considered for any patient with serious infection who demonstrates a poor clinical response to apparently appropriate therapy.

TABLE 18-12. DOSAGES OF IV AND IM ANTIBIOTICS FOR SERIOUS INFECTIONS IN INFANTS AND CHILDREN

Antibiotic (Trade Name)	Daily Dosage
Aminoglycosides	
Amikacin (Amikin)	22 mg/kg div q8h
Gentamicin (numerous trade names)	7.5 mg/kg div q8h
Kanamycin (Kantrex, Klebcil)	30 mg/kg div q8h
Netilmicin (Netromycin)	7.5 mg/kg div q8h
Streptomycin	20 mg/kg div q12h
Tobramycin (Nebcin)	5 mg/kg div q8h
Cephalosporins	
Cefamandole (Mandol)	150 mg/kg div q6h
Cefazolin (Ancef, Kefzol)	100 mg/kg div q8h
Cefoperazone (Cefobid)	(>12 yr) 150 mg/kg div q8h
Cefotaxime (Claforan)	200 mg/kg div q6h
Cefoxitin (Mefoxin)	150 mg/kg div q6h
Ceftazidime (Fortaz, Tazidime)	100–150 mg/kg div q8h
Ceftizoxime (Cefizox)	(>6 mo) 200 mg/kg div q6h
Ceftriaxone (Rocephin)	100 mg/kg div q12h
Cefuroxime (Zinacef)	150 mg/kg div q8h
Cephalothin (Keflin)	100 mg/kg div q6h
Cephapirin (Cefadyl)	75 mg/kg div q6h
Cephradine (Anspor, Velosef)	100 mg/kg div q6h
Moxalactam (Moxam)	200 mg/kg div q6h
Chloramphenicol (Chloromycetin)	100 mg/kg div q6h
Clindamycin (Cleocin)	40 mg/kg div q6h
Erythromycin (numerous trade names)	40 mg/kg div q6h
Lincomycin (Lincocin)	20 mg/kg div q8h

(continued)

TABLE 18-12. (continued)

Antibiotic (Trade Name)	Daily Dosage
Metronidazole (Flagyl)	30 mg/kg div q6h
Penicillins	
Penicillin G	400,000 U/kg div q6h
Penicillin G, benzathine (IM)	50,000 U/kg single dose (IM)
Penicillin G, procaine (IM)	50,000 U/kg div q12h (IM)
Ampicillin (numerous trade names)	200 mg/kg div q6h
Carbenicillin (Geopen, Pyopen)	400 mg/kg div q6h
Methicillin (Celbenin, Staphcillin)	200 mg/kg div q6h
Mezlocillin (Mezlin)	200 mg/kg div q6h
Nafcillin (Nafcil, Unipen)	200 mg/kg div q6h
Oxacillin (Bactocill, Prostaphlin)	200 mg/kg div q6h
Ticarcillin (Ticar)	300 mg/kg div q6h
Streptomycin (IM)	30 mg/kg div q12h (IM)
Sulfonamides	
Sulfadiazine	100 mg/kg div q6h
Sulfisoxazole	100 mg/kg div q6h
Tetracyclines	
Doxycycline (numerous trade names)	5 mg/kg div q24h
Minocycline (Minocin)	4 mg/kg div q12h
Tetracycline (numerous trade names)	25 mg/kg div q8h
Vancomycin (Vancocin)	40 mg/kg div q6h

For the three most common minor infections requiring antibiotic therapy, i.e., otitis media, streptococcal pharyngitis, and skin infections, a maximum dosage of 1 g of a penicillin, cephalosporin, or erythromycin is recommended. In the case of ampicillin, this maximum dosage is reached as early as 10 kg or 1 year of age.

Dosage calculations need not be exact but calculated so that a convenient individual dose is prescribed (½ teaspoon, 1 teaspoon, etc.). Whenever possible bid or tid rather than qid dosing intervals should be used because this is more realistic for patient's and parent's nighttime compliance.

TABLE 18-13. DOSAGES OF ORAL ANTIBIOTICS FOR INFANTS AND CHILDREN

Antibiotic (Trade Name)	Daily Dosage
Cephalosporins	
Cefaclor (Ceclor)	50 mg/kg div q8h
Cefadroxil (Duricef, Ultracef)	30 mg/kg div q12h
Cephalexin (Keflex)	25–50 mg/kg div q6h
Cephradine (Anspor, Velosef)	25–50 mg/kg div q6h
Chloramphenicol	50–100 mg/kg div q6h
Clindamycin (Cleocin)	25 mg/kg div q6h
Colistin (Coly-Mycin)	5–15 mg/kg div q8h
Erythromycin (numerous trade names)	25–50 mg/kg div q6h
Erythromycin and sulfisoxazole (Pediazole)	25–50 mg/kg of erythromycin div q6h
Isoniazid (INH, Nydrazid)	10–30 mg/kg div q12h
Methenamine mandelate (Mandelamine, Thiacide, Uroquid)	50 mg/kg div q6h
Metronidazole (Flagyl, Metryl, Protostat, Satric)	25 mg/kg div q8h
Nalidixic acid (NegGram)	50 mg/kg div q6h
Neomycin (Mycifradin, Neobiotic)	50–100 mg/kg div q6h
Nitrofurantoin (Furadantin, Macrodantin)	7 mg/kg div q6h 2 mg/kg div q24h (for urinary tract suppressive therapy)
Penicillins	
Penicillin V (numerous trade names)	< 10 kg, 375 mg div q8h > 10 kg, 750 mg div q8h
Amoxicillin (numerous trade names)	20–40 mg/kg div q8h

(continued)

TABLE 18-13. (continued)

Antibiotic (Trade Name)	Daily Dosage
Ampicillin (numerous trade names)	50–100 mg/kg div q6h
Bacampicillin (Spectrobid)	25–50 mg/kg div q12h
Carbenicillin (Geocillin)	25–50 mg/kg div q6h
Cloxacillin (Tegopen)	50–100 mg/kg div q6h
Cyclacillin (Cyclapen-W)	50–100 mg/kg div q8h
Dicloxacillin (Dycill, Dynapen, Pathocil)	25 mg/kg div q6h
Hetacillin (Versapen)	50–100 mg/kg div q6h
Pyrazinamide	30 mg/kg div q12h
Rifampin (Rifadin, Rimactane)	20 mg/kg div q24h
Sulfonamides	
Sulfadiazine	150 mg/kg div q6h
Sulfamethoxazole (Gantanol)	50 mg/kg div q12h
Sulfisoxazole (Gantrisin, SK-Soxazole)	100–150 mg/kg div q6h
Tetracyclines	
Tetracycline (numerous trade names)	40 mg/kg div q6h
Demeclocycline (Declomycin)	8–12 mg/kg div q6h
Doxycycline (Vibramycin)	5 mg/kg div q12h
Methacycline (Rondomycin)	10 mg/kg div q6h
Minocycline (Minocin)	4 mg/kg div q12h
Oxytetracycline (Terramycin, Urobiotic 250)	40 mg/kg div q6h
TMP-SMX (Bactrim, Septra, Cotrim, Sulfatrim)	6–12 mg TMP/30–60 mg SMX/kg div q12h 4 mg TMP/20 mg SMX/kg div q12h for *Pneumocystis* prophylaxis 20 mg TMP/100 mg SMX/kg div q6h for *Pneumocystis* treatment
Vancomycin (Vancocin) *Note:* this is not absorbed	50 mg/kg div q6h

Maximum (Adult) Dosages

For many antibiotics, maximum dosage limitations are reached by approximately 12 years of age (40 to 50 kg). In these older children, the volume of distribution is decreased thereby increasing the possibility of overdosing and accompanying toxicity if calculations are made by body weight as with younger patients. Maximum dosages of oral antibiotics are reached even earlier in life, and amounts of antibiotic in tablets and capsules (commonly 250 mg and 500 mg) reflect this limitation.

TABLE 18-14. MAXIMUM (ADULT) DOSAGES OF PARENTERAL ANTIBIOTICS

Antibiotic (Trade Name)	Daily Dosage
Aminoglycosides	
Amikacin	1 g
Gentamicin	300 mg
Kanamycin	1 g
Netilmicin	300 mg
Streptomycin	2 g
Tobramycin	300 mg
Cephalosporins	
Cefamandole	6 g
Cefazolin	6 g
Cefoperazone	12 g
Cefotaxime	12 g
Cefoxitin	12 g
Ceftazidime	9 g
Ceftizoxime	12 g
Ceftriaxone	4 g
Cefuroxime	6 g
Cephalothin	12 g
Moxalactam	12 g
Chloramphenicol	6 g
Clindamycin	4 g
Erythromycin	4 g
Metronidazole	4 g
Penicillins	
Penicillin G	24 million U

(*continued*)

TABLE 18–14. (continued)

Antibiotic (Trade Name)	Daily Dosage
Penicillin G, benzathine	2.4 million U
Penicillin G, procaine	4.8 million U
Ampicillin	12 g
Azlocillin	24 g
Carbenicillin	40 g
Methicillin	18 g
Mezlocillin	24 g
Nafcillin	12 g
Oxacillin	12 g
Piperacillin	24 g
Ticarcillin	24 g
Spectinomycin	4 g
Tetracycline	2 g
Vancomycin	4 g

Body Surface Area

Patients who are excessively obese or malnourished will be over-dosed or underdosed, respectively, if antibiotic dosages are calculated by weight. For these patients, body surface area may be determined by the equation included in Chapter 5, p. 125.

TABLE 18–15. DOSAGES OF ANTIBIOTICS BY BODY SURFACE AREA

Antibiotic	Daily Dosage/m^2
Aminoglycosides	
Amikacin	600 mg div q8h
Gentamicin	180 mg div q8h
Kanamycin	600 mg div q8h
Netilmicin	180 mg div q8h
Tobramycin	150 mg div q8h
Cephalosporins	
Cefamandole	3.5 g div q6h
Cefazolin	2.4 g div q8h

TABLE 18–15. (continued)

Antibiotic	Daily Dosage/m^2
Cefotaxime	3.5 g div q8h
Cefuroxime	2.4 g div q8h
Cephalothin	4.5 g div q6h
Moxalactam	3.5 g div q6h
Chloramphenicol	2 g div q6h
Penicillins	
Penicillin G	7.2 million U div q6h
Ampicillin	4.5 g div q6h
Azlocillin	10 g div q6h
Carbenicillin	16 g div q6h
Methicillin	4.5 g div q6h
Mezlocillin	10 g div q6h
Nafcillin	3.5 g div q6h
Oxacillin	4.5 g div q6h
Piperacillin	10 g div q6h
Ticarcillin	10 g div q6h
TMP-AMX	300 mg TMP/1.5 g SMX div q8h
Vancomycin	1.1–1.7 g div q6h

ANTIBIOTICS FOR SPECIFIC PATHOGENS

For many patients, a clinical syndrome is readily apparent at presentation. Pending results of cultures and their antibiotic sensitivities, therapy should be instituted based on reported susceptibility or efficacy data. The following table summarizes recommended initial antimicrobial therapy. Appropriateness of antibiotics should be reevaluated once culture information is available.

TABLE 18–16. THERAPY FOR DEFINED CLINICAL SYNDROMES OR SPECIFIC MICROORGANISMS

Infection	Drug of Choice	Alternatives
Actinomycosis	Penicillin G	Tetracycline
Adenitis (Chap. 4)	Cloxacillin, dicloxacillin,	

(continued)

TABLE 18-16. (continued)

Infection	Drug of Choice	Alternatives
	oxacillin, cephalexin, or erythromycin	
Anthrax	Penicillin	Erythromycin
Bartonellosis	Penicillin	Tetracycline
Botulism (Chap. 1)	Penicillin	Tetracycline
Brucellosis	Streptomycin *PLUS* tetracycline	
Campylobacter enteritis (Chap. 8)	Erythromycin	
Chancroid (Chap. 15)	TMP-SMX or erythromycin	Streptomycin
Chlamydia pneumonia (Chap. 7)	Erythromycin	Sulfisoxazole
Cholera	Tetracycline	
Diphtheria (Chap. 1)	Penicillin	Erythromycin
Endocarditis (Chap. 1)	Penicillin *PLUS* streptomycin	
Erysipelas (Chap. 4)	Penicillin	Erythromycin
Gas gangrene	Penicillin	Tetracycline
Glanders	Streptomycin *PLUS* tetracycline	
Gonorrhea (Chap. 15)	Penicillin, ampicillin, or amoxicillin	Tetracycline spectinomycin, cefoxitin, cefotaxime, or ceftriaxone
Granuloma inguinale (Chap. 15)	Tetracycline	Erythromycin or gentamicin
Impetigo (Chap. 12)	Penicillin	Erythromycin
Legionnaire's disease Chap. 7)	Erythromycin	

TABLE 18-16. (continued)

Infection	Drug of Choice	Alternatives
Leprosy	Clofazimine *PLUS* dapsone *PLUS* rifampin	
Leptospirosis	Penicillin	Tetracycline
Listeriosis	Ampicillin	TMP-SMX
Ludwig's angina (Chap. 12)	Penicillin *PLUS* clindamycin	
Lyme disease	Penicillin	Tetracycline
Melioidosis	Chloramphenicol *PLUS* sulfisoxazole	
Meningococcemia (Chap. 1)	Penicillin	Cefotaxime, ceftriaxone, or moxalactam
Necrotizing fasciitis	Nafcillin *PLUS* cefotaxime, ceftriaxone, or moxalactam	
Nocardiosis	Sulfisoxazole or TMP-SMX	
Otitis externa (Chap. 4)	Antibiotic–steroid ear drops	
Otitis media (Chap. 4)	Amoxicillin	Cefaclor erythromycin-sulfisoxazole
Parotitis, suppurative	Nafcillin *PLUS* gentamicin	
Pertussis (Chap. 7)	Erythromycin	
Plague	Streptomycin *PLUS* tetracycline	Chloramphenicol

(*continued*)

TABLE 18–16. (continued)

Infection	Drug of Choice	Alternatives
Pneumocystis carinii (Chap. 16)	TMP-SMX	Pentamidine
Pseudomembranous colitis (Chap. 8)	Vancomycin PO	Metronidazole or bacitracin
Q fever	Chloramphenicol or tetracycline	
Rat bite fever	Penicillin	Tetracycline
Relapsing fever	Tetracycline or chloramphenicol	
Rickettsialpox	Chloramphenicol or tetracycline	
Salmonellosis (Chap. 8)	Ampicillin, chloramphenicol or TMP-SMX	
Scarlet fever	Penicillin	Erythromycin
Shigellosis (Chap. 8)	TMP-SMX	
Sinusitis (Chap. 7)	Amoxicillin	Cefaclor or erythromycin-sulfa combination
Staphylococcal scalded skin syndrome	Nafcillin (methicillin for neonates)	
Syphilis (Chap. 15)	Penicillin	Tetracycline or erythromycin
Tetanus (Chap. 1)	Penicillin	Tetracycline
Toxic shock syndrome (Chap. 1)	Nafcillin	Cephalothin
Toxoplasmosis (Chap. 2)	Pyrimethamine *PLUS* sulfadiazine	
Traveler's diarrhea (Chap. 8)	TMP-SMX	Doxycycline
Tuberculosis (Chap. 7)	Isoniazid *PLUS* rifampin	
Tularemia	Streptomycin	Gentamicin or tetracycline

TABLE 18–16. (continued)

Infection	Drug of Choice	Alternatives
Typhoid fever	Chloramphenicol	TMP-SMX
Typhus	Chloramphenicol	Tetracycline
Vincent's angina	Penicillin	Erythromycin
Yersinosis	TMP-SMX	Ampicillin or gentamicin

ANTIVIRAL AGENTS

Antiviral therapy of proven efficacy is currently available for the treatment of four viruses: influenza A, herpes simplex type 1, herpes simplex type 2, and varicella-zoster. For herpes group virus infections, therapy is initiated only for certain well-defined infections. Many other antiviral agents are currently under investigation and two, which may be approved in the near future, interferon and ribavirin, are included in the table below.

TABLE 18–17. THERAPY FOR VIRAL INFECTIONS

Organism	Clinical Infection	Therapy
HBV	Chronic	Interferon (investigational)
HSV	Encephalitis and neonatal disease	Acyclovir (Zovirax) IV 30 mg/kg/day div q8h × 10 days
	Genital primary infection	Acyclovir (Zovirax) 5% ointment cover lesions q3h, 6 × a day × 7 days
	Genital, severe primary infection	Acyclovir (Zovirax) IV 15 mg/kg/day div q8h × 5 days
	Keratoconjunctivitis	Trifluridine (Viroptic) 1% solution 1 drop q2h for 7–21 days

(continued)

TABLE 18–17. (continued)

Organism	Clinical Infection	Therapy
		Vidarabine (Vira-A) 3% ointment 5 × a day q3–4h × 7–21 days
	Mucosal and cutaneous infection in immunocompromised patients or neonates	Acyclovir (Zovirax) IV 750 mg/m^2/day div q8h × 7 days
Influenza A	Prophylaxis or pneumonia	Amantadine (Symmetrel) PO 5–8 mg/kg/day div q12h (max 200 mg/day)
Respiratory syncytial virus	Pneumonia	Ribavirin (Virazole) (investigational)
VZV	Progressive cutaneous disease in the immunocompromised host	Vidarabine (Vira-A) IV 10 mg/kg/day div q24h × 5 days or acyclovir IV 30 mg/kg/day div q8h × 5 days

ANTIFUNGAL AGENTS

Systemic fungal infections are being seen with increased frequency as a result of longer survival for patients with severe disease and compromised immune function. Broad spectrum antibiotics and indwelling foreign bodies (central IV lines, urinary catheters, and arterial monitoring catheters) are the most significant predisposing factors, particularly for infection with *Candida albicans*. Therefore, strong consideration must be given for discontinuing these antibiotics and removing any indwelling source for fungal colonization.

Amphotericin B remains the most commonly recommended antifungal agent, yet is perhaps the most toxic antimicrobial agent used in medical practice. Renal function must be carefully monitored and, whenever possible, dosage and duration of therapy should be minimized. Current investigative protocols are examining ketoconazole as a substitute for amphotericin B for the treatment of various systemic mycoses.

TABLE 18-18. THERAPY FOR FUNGAL INFECTIONS

Mycosis	Clinical Infection	Therapy
Aspergillosis	Pulmonary or systemic	Amphotericin B 30 mg/kg total dose
Blastomycosis	Pulmonary, bone, skin, or systemic	Amphotericin B 30 mg/kg total dose
Candidiasis	Thrush or diaper rash	Oral nystatin 200,000 U qid × 6–12 days and nystatin cream qid
	Cystitis	irrigate bladder with amphotericin B 10 mg/100 ml (see Chap. 10); remove catheter
	Systemic infection in the neonate	Amphotericin B 0.5 mg/kg/day IV *PLUS* flucytosine 150 mg/kg/day PO div q6h × 30 days
	Candidemia in the immunocompromised host	Amphotericin B 0.3 −1 mg/kg/day × 14–30 days
	Severe colonization (mouth, esophagus, GI tract) in the immunocompromised host	Ketoconazole in 5–10 mg/kg/day div q12h × 7 days or oral nystatin
Coccidioidomycosis	Pulmonary	Amphotericin B 30 mg/kg total dose
Cryptococcosis	Pulmonary	Amphotericin B 0.3 mg/kg/day IV *PLUS* flucytosine 150 mg/kg/day PO div q6h × 30 days

(continued)

TABLE 18-18. (continued)

Mycosis	Clinical Infection	Therapy
	Meningitis	Amphotericin B 1 mg/kg/day × 30 days or until CSF cryptococcal antigen titer ≤ 1:2
Dermatophytoses	Kerion	Griseofulvin 11 mg/kg/day PO div q24h × 3 wk
	Ringworm or other skin lesions	Griseofulvin PO or topical clotrimazole or miconazole
Histoplasmosis	Progressive pulmonary disease in older children	Amphotericin B 30 mg/kg total dose
	Systemic disease in young infants	1 mg/kg day x 14 days
Phycomycosis (mucormycosis, zygomycosis)	Sinusitis and midline facial infection	Amphotericin B 30 mg/kg total dose
Ringworm (see Dermatophytoses)		
Sporotrichosis	Soft tissue, bone or joint infection	SSKI until infection resolved
	Systemic	Amphotericin B 30 mg/kg total dose

TABLE 18-19. ANTIFUNGAL THERAPY

Agent (Trade Name)	Dosage
Amphotericin B (Fungizone)	1 mg test dose, followed in 4 hr by 0.25 mg/kg IV. Increase dosage each day by 0.25 mg/kg to a maximum of 1

TABLE 18-19. (continued)

Agent (Trade Name)	Dosage
	mg/kg/day given as a single daily infusion. For most systemic infections, a total dose of 30 mg/kg is required When combined with flucytosine, the daily dose is 0.3 mg/kg
Flucytosine (Ancobon)	150 mg/kg day PO div q6h
Griseofulvin (numerous trade names)	11 mg/kg/day PO div q24h
Ketoconazole (Nizoral)	5–10 mg/kg/day PO div q12h
Nystatin (Mycostatin, Nilstat)	200,000 U (2 ml) PO qid × 6–12 days
Saturated solution of potassium iodide (SSKI)	1–2 drops per yr of age, tid, (max 20 drops tid) × 2–6 wk

ANTIPARASITIC AGENTS

Parasitic infections are much less commonly encountered in medical practice as contrasted with just one generation ago. This change is attributed primarily to improved urban sanitation. Moreover, few cities have retained soil conditions necessary for maintenance of the life cycle of most parasites. Pinworms remain the most common parasitic infestation seen in the United States and therapy is usually not indicated since recurrence is almost universal. Giardiasis is being seen with greater frequency as a result of increased use of day-care centers where disease is readily transmitted.

For unusual parasitic infections, telephone consultation should be obtained from the Centers for Disease Control, Atlanta, Ga., where many of the preferred therapeutic agents are available. The daytime number is 404–329–3670; the night or weekend number is 404–329–3644.

TABLE 18–20. THERAPY FOR COMMON PARASITIC INFECTIONS

Disease/Parasite	Therapy
Amebiasis *Entamoeba histolytica*	
Asymptomatic or intestinal	Iodoquinol (Yodoxin) 40 mg/kg/day PO div q8h × 20 days *PLUS* metronidazole (Flagyl, Metryl) 40 mg/kg/day PO div q8h × 10 days *OR* paromomycin (Humatin) 30 mg/kg/day PO div q8h × 10 days
Hepatic	Iodoquinol + metronidazole as above *OR* iodoquinol + dehydroemetine (obtain from CDC) 1–1.5 mg/kg/day IM div q12h × 5 days (max 90 mg/day) *FOLLOWED BY* chloroquine (Aralen) 10 mg/kg/day (max 600 mg/day) PO div q8h × 21 days
Ascariasis *Ascaris lumbricoides*	Mebendazole (Vermox) 1 tab bid × 3 days *OR* pyrantel pamoate (Antiminth) 11 mg/kg PO × one dose *OR* piperazine (Antepar) 75 mg/kg PO daily × 2
Cutaneous larva migrans *Necator americanus* *Ancylostoma duodenale*	Topical thiabendazole (Mintezol) susp div q12h × 5 days
Dientamoeba *Dientamoeba fragilis*	Iodoquinol (Yodoxin) 40 mg/kg/day PO div q8h × 20 days *OR* tetracycline 40 mg/kg/day PO div q8h × 10 days
Giardiasis *Giardia lamblia*	Metronidazole (Flagyl, Metryl) 25 mg/kg/day PO div q8h × 7 days *OR* furazolidone (Furoxone) 8 mg/kg/day PO div q6h × 10 days
Hookworm *Necator americanus* *Ancylostoma duodenale*	Mebendazole (Vermox) 1 tab bid × 3 days *OR* pyrantel pamoate (Antiminth) 11 mg/kg × one dose
Lice	Shampoo hair with 1% gamma

TABLE 18-20. (continued)

Disease/Parasite	Therapy
Pediculus humanis	benzene hexachloride (Kwell), rinse and repeat in 24 hr
Phthirus pubis	Apply 1% gamma benzene hexachloride (Kwell) to all skin from the neck down for 12 hr
Malaria *Plasmodium vivax* *Plasmodium ovale*	Chloroquine (Aralen) 10 mg base/kg PO followed by 5 mg base/kg 6 hr, 24 hr, and 48 hr after initial dose, *PLUS* primaquine 0.3 mg base/kg PO qd × 14 days
Plasmodium malariae	Chloroquine (as above) as single agent
P. falciparum	(Consult CDC as therapy varies according to susceptibility patterns for each geographic region)
Pinworms *Enterobius vermicularis*	Pyrantel pamoate (Antiminth) 11 mg/kg PO daily × 2 *or* mebendazole (Vermox) 1 tablet
Pneumocystis pneumonia *Pneumocystis carinii*	(See Table 17–16)
Scabies *Sarcoptes scabiei*	< 2 yr use 10% crotamiton cream (Eurax) >2 yr 1% gamma benzene hexachloride (Kwell) apply to body below chin at night; wash off in morning; repeat in 24 hr
Strongyloidiasis *Strongyloides stercoralis*	Thiabendazole (Mintezol) 50 mg/kg/day PO div q12h × 2 days
Trichomoniasis *Trichomonas vaginalis*	Metronidazole 15 mg/kg/day PO div q8h × 10 days; for adolescents and adults: single 2 g dose; treat sexual partners
Whipworm *Trichuris trichiura*	Mebendazole (Vermox) 1 tab PO bid × 3 days

APPENDIX:
Definition of Terms and Abbreviations

ABG	arterial blood gases
ADH	antidiuretic hormone
ANA	antinuclear antibody
APPG	aqueous procaine penicillin G
ARDS	adult respiratory distress syndrome
ARF	acute rheumatic fever
ASO	antistreptolysin O
BCG	bacille Calmette-Guérin
CDC	Centers for Disease Control
CF	complement fixation
CHF	congestive heart failure
CIE	counterimmunoelectrophoresis
CMV	cytomegalovirus
CoA	coagglutination
CPAP	continuous positive airway pressure
CRP	C-reactive protein
CT	computed tomography
CVA	cardiovascular accident
CVP	central venous pressure
DGI	disseminated gonococcal infection
DIC	disseminated intravascular coagulation
EBV	Epstein-Barr virus
ELISA	enzyme linked immunosorbent assay
EMB	eosin methylene blue
ESR	erythrocyte sedimentation rate
ETEC	enterotoxigenic *Escherichia coli*

EOM	extraocular movements
FA	fluorescent antibody
FTA-abs	fluorescent *Treponema* antibody-absorbed
FUO	fever of unknown origin
GBS	Guillain-Barré syndrome
GC	gonococcal
HAV	hepatitis A virus
HBV	hepatitis B virus
HDCV	human diploid cell vaccine
HI	hemagglutination inhibition
HRIG	human rabies immune globulin
HSV	herpes simplex virus
IFA	indirect fluorescent antibody
IHA	indirect hemagglutination
IHSS	idiopathic hypertrophic subaortic stenosis
INH	isoniazid
IPPB	intermittent positive pressure breathing
IUG	intrauterine growth retardation
IUD	intrauterine device
JRA	juvenile rheumatoid arthritis
LA	left atrium
LGV	*Lymphogranuloma venereum*
LTB	laryngotracheobronchitis
LV	left ventrical
LVH	left ventricular hypertrophy
MBC	minimum bactericidal concentration
MDM	minor determinant mixture
MHA-TP	microhemagglutination-*Treponema pallidum*
MIC	minimum inhibitory concentration
MMR	measles, mumps, rubella (vaccine)
NEC	necrotizing enterocolitis
NG	nasogastric
NGU	nongonoccocal urethritis
NMR	nuclear magnetic resonance
PCWP	pulmonary capillary wedge pressure
PDA	patent ductus arteriosis
PEEP	positive end expiratory pressure

PHA	phytohemagglutinin
PID	pelvic inflammatory disease
PMC	Pseudomembranous colitis
PMN	polymorphonuclear
PPD	purified protein derivative
PPL	penicilloyl polylysine
PPNG	penicillinase producing *Neisseria gonorrhoeae*
PT	prothrombin time
RA	right atrium
RIA	radioimmunoassay
RMSF	Rocky Mountain spotted fever
RSV	respiratory syncytial virus
SCID	severe combined immunodeficiency
SF	synovial fluid
SG	specific gravity
SIADH	syndrome of inappropriate antidiuretic hormone
SKSD	streptokinase-streptodornase
SLE	systemic lupus erythematosus
SS	salmonella-shigella
SSKI	saturated solution of potassium iodide
STD	sexually transmitted disease
Td	adult tetanus-diphtheria
TMP-SMX	trimethoprim/sulfamethoxazole
TORCH	toxoplasma, rubella, cytomegalovirus, and herpes simplex
TSA	trypticase soy agar
TSS	toxic shock syndrome
VCUG	voiding cystourethrogram
VDRL	venereal disease research laboratory
VZIG	varicella zoster immune globulin
VZV	varicella zoster virus

Index